Understanding Skin Cancer: A Guide to Basal Cell, Squamous Cell, and Melanoma

Chopra

Contents

1 Introduction   **1**

   1.1 Motivation 1

   1.2 Objectives 2

   1.3 Organization of the work 3

2 Skin cancer   **5**

   2.1 Dermatology 5

   2.2 Teledermatology 7

   2.3 Skin Cancer 8

     2.3.1 Types of skin cancer 8

     2.3.2 Screening for skin cancer 12

    2.3.3   Drawbacks of screening for skin cancer 13

  2.4   Skin cancer data sets 14

3 Literature review 21

  3.1   Background on machine learning 21

      3.1.1   Classifiers 22

      3.1.2   Deep learning 24

      3.1.3   Validation methods and evaluation 26

  3.2   Computer-Aided Diagnosis systems for skin cancer classification 28

      3.2.1   Pre-processing 30

      3.2.2   Segmentation 30

      3.2.3   Feature extraction and selection 31

      3.2.4   Classifiers 32

      3.2.5   Multimodality 33

  3.3   Summary 35

4 Experimental Methodology 37

  4.1   Dataset 37

  4.2   Data pre-processing, augmentation and balancing 39

  4.3   Investigated techniques 42

  4.4   Architecture 42

  4.5   Evaluation metrics 45

  4.6   Experiments 46

      4.6.1   Img: Clinical/Dermoscopic Image (exp1) 47

      4.6.2   ImgMd_CF: Clinical/Dermoscopic Image and Metadata Class-Fusion (exp2) 47

      4.6.3   Img_MT7pts: Clinical/Dermoscopic Image Multitask 7-points (exp3) . . 48

      4.6.4   ImgMd_CF_TransfL7pts: Clinical/Dermoscopic Image and Metadata Class-Fusion with Transfer Learning of multitask 7-points pre-training (exp4) 48

      4.6.5   Img_MtMd: Clinical/Dermoscopic Image Multitask Metadata (exp5) . . 49

4.6.6   ImgMd_CF_TransfLMd: Clinical/Dermoscopic Image and Metadata Class-Fusion with Transfer Learning of multitask Metadata pre-train (exp6) ... 50

4.6.7   ImgMd_FF: Clinical/Dermoscopic Image and Metadata Feature-Fusion (exp7) ... 50

4.6.8   ImgMd_FF_MT7pts: Clinical/Dermoscopic Image and Metadata Feature-Fusion Multitasking 7-points (exp8) ... 51

4.6.9   2Img_FF_MT7pts: Both Images Feature-Fusion Multitasking 7-points (exp9) ... 51

4.6.10 2ImgMd_FF_MT7pts: Both Images Metadata Feature-Fusion Multitasking 7-points (exp10) ... 52

4.6.11 2ImgMd_CombFF_MT7pts: Both Images Metadata Combinations of Feature-Fusion Multitasking 7-points (exp11) ... 53

5   Results and analysis   57

5.1   Hyperparameters ... 57

5.2   Img (exp1) ... 59

5.3   ImgMd_CF (exp2) ... 64

5.4   Img_MT7pts (exp3) ... 66

5.5   ImgMd_CF_TransfL7pts (exp4) ... 67

5.6   Img_MTMd (exp5) ... 70

5.7   ImgMd_CF_TransfLMd (exp6) ... 72

5.8   ImgMd_FF (exp7) ... 75

5.9   ImgMd_FF_MT7pts (exp8) ... 77

5.10 2Img_FF_MT7pts (exp9) ... 80

5.11 2ImgMd_FF_MT7pts (exp10) ... 82

5.12 2ImgMd_CombFF_MT7pts (exp11) ... 83

5.12.1 Single image ... 84

5.12.2 Single Image and Metadata ... 85

5.12.3 Clinical Image, Dermoscopic image and Metadata ... 88

5.13 Summary ... 89

5.13.1 Baseline 89

5.13.2 Class-fusion and feature-fusion. 90

5.13.3 Multitasking 90

5.13.4 Multitasking and multimodality 90

5.13.5 Multitasking and all modalities 90

6 Conclusion   **93**

6.1 Conclusions 93

Chapter 1

Introduction

This chapter provides an introduction to this work. The motivation is explained in Section 1.1. The objectives this work intends to achieve are laid out in Section 1.2. Lastly, the organization of this work is shown in Section 1.3.

1.1 Motivation

Cancer is a dangerous disease with a high mortality rate when diagnosed at later stages. When it comes to skin cancer, there exist a variety of different types. Designated after the cell that originated the cancer, Basal Cell Carcinoma (BCC) and Squamous Cell Carcinoma are the first and second most common skin cancers respectively, while Melanoma is among the most dangerous skin cancers. Skin cancer has been consistently rising in these last few years, with cases of Melanoma predicted to rise from 287,723 in 2018 to 340,271 in 2025 [55]. In Portugal alone, there are over nine thousand cases of Basal Cell Carcinoma and two thousand cases of Squamous Cell Carcinoma [21], while Melanoma has one thousand cases [20].

Melanoma is given more attention due to the considerable danger it presents. Melanoma often spreads to the lymph nodes [62], being then able to spread faster to other parts of the body. While the estimated five-year survival rate from Melanoma when detected early is about 99%, the survival rate falls to 65% when the disease reaches the lymph nodes and 25% when the disease metastasizes to distant organs [26].

There has been a rise in the number of specialists (Dermatologists), however, in the United States, the number remains insufficient to provide adequate care for the general population [32]. With dermatologists also being called upon to take care of many other skin conditions, a solution is needed to address the rising number of skin cancers and insufficient number of dermatologists.

Screening has been used to attempt to identify cancerous lesions at an early stage, or before symptoms manifest, while methods based on common characteristics observed in previous cancers have been proposed and adopted. However, the screening process is time consuming, while the classification of a lesion as cancerous remains mostly dependent on the dermatologist expertise.

With the classification process being largely visual, images are usually taken. Computer-Aided Diagnosis (CAD) systems that aid in the classification of skin cancers have been under investigation since 1987 [52]. These usually take the obtained images as input to predict a classification. Advances in technology have enabled the easier adoption of a dermatoscope, a device that enables the capture of dermoscopic images. As usually only dermatologists use dermatoscopes, clinical (macroscopic) images are still taken and kept on the medical records. Regardless, despite dermoscopic images being cleaner and having a higher level of detail than a clinical image, clinical images still contain relevant information. Even dermatologists obtain better results when they have access to various modalities such as dermoscopic images, clinical images and metadata, [35], however research on CAD systems that utilize multiple modalities is small in comparison with the larger research on CAD systems.

Recent developments have shown that deep learning is a promising technology, having surpassed human performance in visual tasks such as playing Atari games, board games like Go and object recognition [24]. This technology has been integrated in various CAD systems, obtaining comparable results to more classical.

1.2   Objectives

This thesis was developed in Fraunhofer Portugal in collaboration with Sciences Faculty of University of Porto. This work is part of project "DERM.AI: Usage of Artificial Intelligence to Power Teledermatological Screening", with reference DSAIPA/AI/0031/2018, and supported by national funds through 'FCT—Foundation for Science and Technology, I.P.'. Derm.AI project aims to contribute to processes optimization between Primary Care Units and Dermatology Services of the National Health Service, namely through the integration of a mobile application to acquire macroscopic skin lesion images and the development of AI-powered Risk Prioritization and Decision Support platform.

To support this project, this work studies the classification of skin cancer lesions using multiple modalities from the domain. The impact of using each modality, or a combination of them, to the quality of the lesion classification is investigated. Several techniques are investigated regarding their efficacy in improving the results obtained from fusing the modalities. The effects of using a simple architecture are also investigated, determining its viability. As various tests are performed, the simple architecture also facilitate a faster testing of these various subjects (modalities and techniques). Lastly, this work is heavily influenced by the work in [44], where, in addition to multitasking, several combinations of modalities are performed in the same model. This methodology is adapted and investigated. These objectives can be summarised in the following points:

1. Investigate the impact of each modality to the quality of the skin cancer classification.

2. Investigate the impact of the fusion of the modalities in the quality of the skin cancer classification.

3. Investigate the impact of several techniques to the quality of the skin cancer classification.

4. Determine the viability of a simple architecture in skin cancer classification.

5. Investigate the impact of performing several combinations of modalities on the same model.

1.3 Organization of the work

This work is made up of six chapters. This first chapter is the introduction to the work. The following two chapters provide further context, with Chapter 2 providing a full description of dermatology, skin cancer, screening and the available datasets. Chapter 3 contains a review of the state of the art regarding CAD systems. Topics such as machine learning and deep learning are introduced and explained in this chapter, followed by an overview of the methods utilized in various CAD systems with a focus works with multimodality. A set of experiments was designed to study various aspects of lesion classification using single modality and multiple modalities. The methodology and rationale for these experiments are presented in Chapter 4. Results are described, analysed and discussed in Chapter 5. Finally, Chapter 6 concludes this work and presents perspectives of future work.

Chapter 2

Skin cancer

This chapter introduces main concepts related with dermatology and skin cancer. Beginning with defining the terminology used in dermatology in Section 2.1 and teledermatology in Section 2.2. The most important skin cancers are described and the most common benign lesions are explained in Section 2.3. Screening is explained in Sub-Section 2.3.2 with the available datasets being briefly described and summarized in Section 2.4.

2.1   Dermatology

Dermatology is the field of medicine specialised in the management of skin conditions. The skin is the largest organ of the body, being composed by three layers, the epidermis, dermis and hypodermis.

The epidermis is the outermost layer of the skin, it houses cells such as squamous, basal, melanocytes and merkel cells, among others. Its job is to protect the body from the environment. The dermis stands below the epidermis layer, containing tough connective tissue, hair follicles, and sweat glands. While the deepest layer, hypodermis, is made of fat and connective tissue, functioning as an insulator and shock-absorber [61].

The scope of dermatology involves all kinds of skin conditions, from cosmetic applications to inflammatory, inherited, environmental, occupational and malignant skin diseases. Its specialists are the dermatologists. Their patients belong to all ages and sexes, and while some injuries require assistance, most of the time the patients will not stay overnight at the hospital (outpatients) [37]. Usually, the patients are redirected to a dermatologist by a general practitioner when suspicious skin lesions are found during a consultation.

Of the many conditions that dermatology oversees, skin cancer is one of the most dangerous. Depending on the situation, the treatment can range from chemotherapy to a biopsy, an operation where the affected part is removed. If the cancer is not diagnosed and treated in time, it will spread through the body (metastasis), resulting in the eventual passing of the patient.

Similar to other types of cancer, it is of great importance to confirm and accurately classify the cancer type. Early detection of cancer increases the chances of survival and reduces the morbidity and cost of the treatment [84]. When compared with other types of cancer, skin cancer has the inherent advantage of being directly visible in the body. Although this fact leads to easier detection and treatment of the lesion, it comes with its own obstacles. The skin, as the barrier between the inside and outside of the body, is home to many types of lesions. Most result from outside trauma, such as scratches, cuts or bruises. Some are benign and entirely cosmetic in nature, such as scars. Others are benign but can evolve into malignant lesions, such as moles. Malignant lesions can be divided into multiple categories such as cancers or warts, each having further specific subcategories.

The main problem in skin cancer is the confirmation of a lesion as cancerous, as the appearance of skin cancer can vary wildly. Dermatologist need to rely on their years of experience to provide a reliable diagnostic. Scoring systems and methods have been introduced that improve the diagnostic performance of less experienced clinicians [52]. However, these do not reach the desired goal of removing experience from the equation, as these do not raise the performance of a doctor to that of an experienced dermatologists, especially in rare cases. Biopsy is the test performed to obtain a reliable diagnosis, however the test is intrusive.

The usual method to distinguish a malignant lesion (cancer) from a benign lesion is to perform what has been denominated as "Pattern analysis" [68] were a dermatologist matches the traits of the lesion with previously recorded instances, attempting to classify the lesion accordingly [11]. From this practice came the discovery of reoccurring patterns, which led to the creation of several methods that streamline the classification process:

- ABCD rule [18] which consists of the analysis of four criteria, Asymmetry, Border irregularity, Color variegation and Dermoscopic (or Differential) structures, with a semi-quantitative score system. Often the D criteria is used to refer to the size of the lesion, with a lesion with Diameter larger than 6mm being an indication of cancer [1]. The ABCD score is computed as the weighted sum of the category scores. The final score varies from 1 to 8.9. Scores below 4.75 are identified as benign, from 4.75 to 5.45 as a sign of early melanoma, and above 5.45 classified as melanoma.

- ABCDE rule [1], same as above but has in consideration as well the Evolution of a lesion. A lesion is evolving when it changes its size, shape, symptoms (eg, itching, tenderness), surface (eg, bleeding), or shades of color.

- 7-point checklist [5] derived from the analysis of pigmented skin lesions, where 7 criteria, 3 major and 4 minor, are identified. The major criteria have a score value of 2 while the minor have a value of 1. A minimum of 3 total score is needed to identify malignant melanoma.

  The criteria include Atypical pigment network, Blue-white veil, Atypical vascular pattern, as the majors, and Irregular streaks, Irregular pigmentation, Irregular dots/globules and Regression structures, as the minors.

- Menzies method [11], where there are a set of features, 2 negatives and 9 positives. In this method, a lesion is not classified as melanoma if it does not contain any of the negative features and it contains at least one of the positive.

  The negative features consist of point and axial symmetry of pigmentation and presence of a single color, with the positive being blue-white veil, multiple brown dots, pseudopods, radial streaming, scar-like depigmentation, peripheral black dots-globules, multiple colors (5 or 6), Multiple blue/gray dots and broadened network.

Another attempt to streamline the classification process is teledermatology.

2.2 Teledermatology

Teledermatology [49] is the provision of dermatology services without the need to consult a dermatologist in person. This procedure exists thanks to improvements and a higher ease of access to technologies such as the internet and dermatoscopes, as well as the average cameras being able to obtain higher quality images.

With improvements to the camera and dermatoscopes, an average camera can be extended by a simple dermatoscope. This makes it able to capture images of a worrying skin lesion with dermoscopic-like quality. These images, along with a description, are sent through the internet to a queue. The queue is processed by teleconsultants (that are dermatologists). They determine if the lesion requires immediate attention, if the data is inconclusive or if it is benign. This feedback is given typically within a 24 hour period [49].

This method brings several advantages. An immediate opinion is not required, allowing specialists time to verify their conclusion. Despite usually taking 24 hours to provide a response, it is a significant improvement to the current wait time to see a dermatologist. Lastly, this procedure allows access to dermatology care in remote regions where an expert might not be available.

Despite these advantages, there has not been a consensus if teledermatology is comparable to dermatology. However, at its lowest point, it provided results slightly inferior to those of dermatology [49]. These results indicate that teledermatology is a viable way to streamline the triage of patients, ensuring the most urgent ones get treatment sooner. This improves the efficiency of the work time of the dermatologists, as the healthier patients will not necessitate a physical consultation.

A sub field of teledermatology is its mobile variant, where thanks to the improvement of mobile phone cameras, images with increased quality can be acquired by the average person. With use of a simple apparatus, a person can turn a mobile phone into an ad-hoc dermoscopic camera, further streamlining the teledermatology process and making it easier for a patients to provide dermoscopic-like images for check-ups. This is especially beneficial for patients that have past history of skin cancer. They can better monitor a recurrent cancer [12].

Pilot study participants of this sub-procedure report that it is easy to perform and they felt motivated to monitor their skin more often. Barriers to this procedure included the difficulty to reach lesions in some places and the inadequate education of an average person about what lesions are worthy of attention [49].

A lesion can be classified into several types of skin cancer. Identifying the type of skin cancer is important as its danger is it tied to its type. Although all types of skin cancer can progress to more dangerous stages, some progress at a faster pace. A higher skin cancer stage complicates the treatment, leading to an increased cost and a larger impact on the lifestyle of the patient.

2.3 Skin Cancer

It is normal for damage to occur in cells. When such is the case and the damage can not be repaired, cells activate mechanisms to replace themselves. Cancer occurs when the mechanisms themselves are damaged. This causes the cells to not be able to terminate themselves, resulting in them starting to multiply without control [26]. This replication causes an unusual growth in the area, sometimes causing the area to be raised, as well as oozing or bleeding more easily [63]. This effect can be observed in Figure 2.1, it is a graphical representation of the effects of various cancers on the skin. The worst case occurs when the cancerous cells start spreading throughout the body (metastasis), leading to the creation of more cancerous spots and resulting in the eventual death of the patient.

Other factors that cause damage to the skin, particularly damage that can lead to cancer, is exposure to UV radiation (Sun), errors in the genetic code of the cell or usage of tanning beds [26]. A weakened immune system can also increase the risk of skin cancer [63].

2.3.1 Types of skin cancer

Skin cancer type varies from cell to cell, as such, many of their classifications are named after the cell they originate from. Due to the large variety of cells in the skin, there exists a large range of possible skin cancers, with the most common or dangerous types being the following:

- Basal Cell Carcinoma (BCC), most common. (Figure 2.2)

  It is the most common type of skin cancer, covering over 80% of skin cancer classifications, it originates from basal cells, in the lowest part of the epidermis. The basal cell is a cell responsible for producing new skin cell as old ones die off, acting as a regenerative layer for the skin [54]. This cancer tends to occur in areas where the skin is regularly exposed to the sun. Its growth is usually slow, with it being rare to metastasize or spread to nearby lymph nodes, a small bean-shaped structure that is part of the body's immune system [39], but will happen with time.

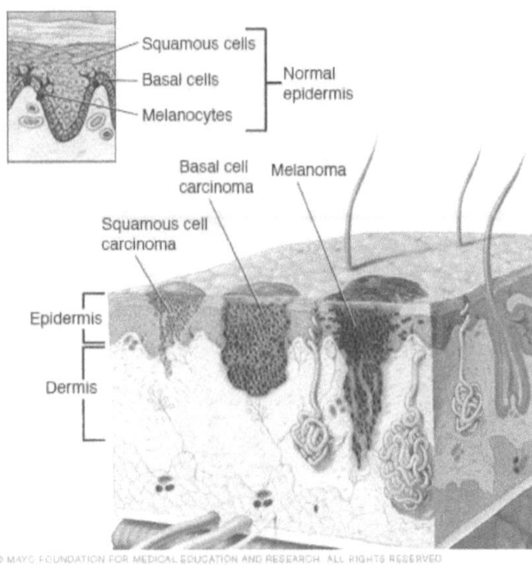

Figure 2.1: Demonstration of various types of cancerous growths on the skin and its layers [54]

BCC has a tendency to reappear/reoccur in the same location after being successfully treated/removed with a 50% chance of recurrence within five years of the first diagnosis [63]. Several features can be recognized in the cancerous region, such as open sores, red patches, pink growths, shiny bumps, scars or growths with slightly elevated, rolled edges and/or a central indentation which, at times, may ooze, crust, itch or bleed. In patients with darker skin, about half of BCCs are pigmented (meaning brown in color). BCCs can vary significantly from person to person [26].

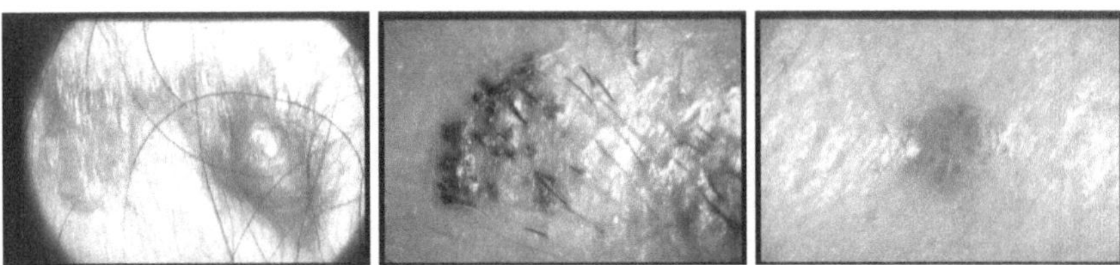

Figure 2.2: Examples of Basal Cell Carcinoma [4]

- Squamous Cell Carcinoma (SCC), second most common.

  The Second most common type of skin cancer, develops at the flat, thin squamous cells that make up much of epidermis, the outermost layer of the skin [63]. Squamous cells are found in many places of the body [54], occurring commonly in places where absorption or transportation of materials plays an important role such as in diffusion, osmosis and filtration [10].

Like BCC, the cancer typically occurs in places that have been exposed to the sun, but may develop in other areas that contain scars or skin ulcers, as well as in the genital region. Some characteristics, like the slow growth and difficulty spreading or metastasizing, are also shared with BCC, however SCC has higher chances to invade fatty tissue beneath the skin or spread even further [63]. It occurs with features like scaly red patches, open sores, rough, thickened or wart-like skin, or raised growths with a central depression. SCCs may, at times, crust over, itch or bleed, with its features varying from person to person [26].

- Melanoma, most dangerous. (Figure 2.3)

Melanoma is the most serious type of skin cancer, developing from melanocytes, a cell found in the epidermis. The melanocytes is a cell responsible for the production of melanin, a pigment responsible for the color of the skin [26]. These cells darken when exposed to the sun, shielding the deeper layers of the skin from the harmful effects of the ultraviolet (UV) rays from the sun [63]. Since it forms from melanocytes, it usually occurs in the skin, regardless if it is exposed to the sun, but can also appear on the eyes and, rarely, in internal organs, such as the intestines. The exact cause is not clear, but exposure to UV radiation from sunlight or tanning lamps and beds increases the risk of developing melanoma [54].

Contrary to BCC and SCC, melanoma tends to spread to other parts of the body. The cancerous cells are often found in lymph nodes, being able to spread via the lymphatic channels, which connect other lymph nodes throughout the body [62]. It can occur with different shapes, sizes and colors. Due to this it is hard to provide an easy guide for identification to inexperienced people. Despite this, they typically either mutate from existing moles, $20 - 30\%$, or form mole-like lesions on normal skin, $70 - 80\%$ [26].

Melanoma can be sub-categorized in several sub-types of malignant melanoma. The superficial spreading melanoma, nodular melanoma and lentigo maligna melanomas make up to 90% of all diagnosed malignant melanomas. The remaining 10% are filled by the rarer types such as acral lentiginous melanoma and acral amelanotic malignant melanoma [62]. Each sub-type of melanoma has its own features, some being extremely different from other. The superficial spreading malignant melanoma occurs as a new or a mutation from an existing mole, while nodular malignant melanoma takes a blue or red appearance, typically occurring as a new mole.

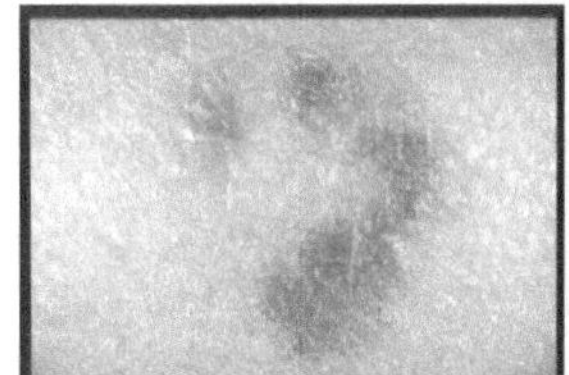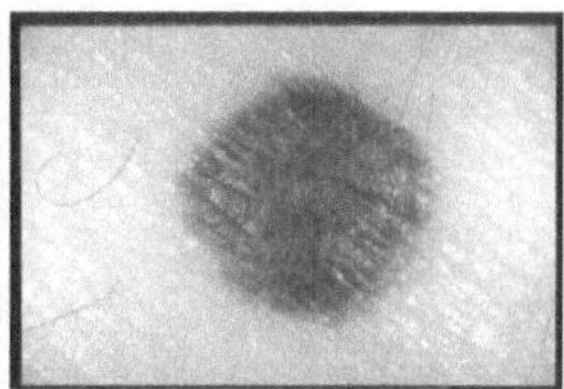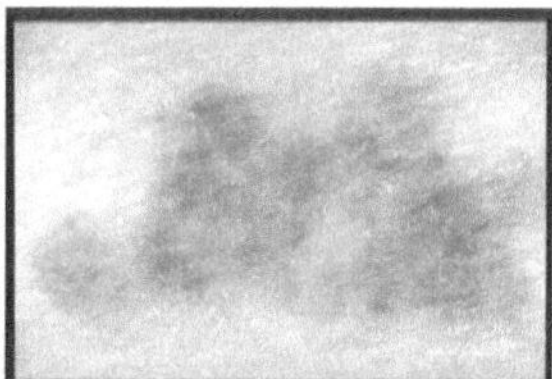

Figure 2.3: Examples of Melanoma [4]

- Merkel Cell Carcinoma (MCC), rarer but dangerous

  This is a rarer type of skin cancer but equally as dangerous as melanoma, with it forming from Merkel cells, in the epidermis layer of the skin [58, 63]. Merkel cells provide, along with nerve endings, the sense of touch from the skin [63].

  MCC appears more commonly in areas of the skin exposed to the sun, as well as in people with age over 50 and weakened immune system. Like melanoma, MCC is an aggressive form of skin cancer with a high risk of recurring and metastasizing, often within two to three years after initial diagnosis [26]. It frequently targets the brain, bones, liver and lungs when it metastasizes [63].

  MCC is harder to find than other skin cancers, as it can appear as a pearly pimple-like lump, sometimes skin-colored, red, purple or bluish-red, though they are rarely tender to the touch. Often patients and doctors only discover the cancerous formation due to its alarmingly high rate of growth [26].

  It is worth noting that Merkel Cell Carcinoma was denominated after the Merkel cell due to the similarities between the cells. However, since said cell does not self-replicate, the cancerous cells derive from the progenitor, usually epidermal precursor cells [58].

There are various medical terms that describe/encompass various types of cancer. The easiest to understand is the "non-melanoma cancer". Due to the danger and frequency of melanoma, all other types of cancer can be classified under non-melanoma cancers. Another term is the "keratinocyte carcinomas" that includes cancers originating from cells birthed from a cell called keratinocyte, BCC and SCC cancers belong in this group [64].

Cancerous cells are not the only thing a doctor should be on guard for. As cancer can develop in previously healthy lesions, some lesions should be paid attention to, either for their close resemblance to a cancer, or because they have a high likelihood to become cancerous. The Seborrheic Keratosis (SK) (Figure 2.4) is a common benign skin growth. The factors that lead to its occurrence are not well known, but they tend to occur in people older than 50 and within families, so genes are believed to play a role [54]. Generally harmless and not contagious, treatment is not necessary, however clothing can cause them to irritate or bleed. Otherwise, if signs such as sores, quick increase in size, bleeding and not healing appear, it usually indicates the development of cancer [54]. Typically appearing on the head, neck, chest or back, multiple growths are common, with their appearance being usually brown, black or light tan, with a waxy, scaly and slightly raised look [54].

Nevus (NEV) (Figure 2.5) is another benign skin lesion. Nevi (plural) is the medical term used for various skin formations such as moles, birthmarks or beauty marks. A common occurrence, nevi is a collection of harmless colored cells, typically appearing as a small brown, tan, or pink spots [65]. A person can both be born with these or develop new ones later.

The later a skin cancer is diagnosed, the harder the treatment, as such, screening has been used as an attempt to identify skin cancer early.

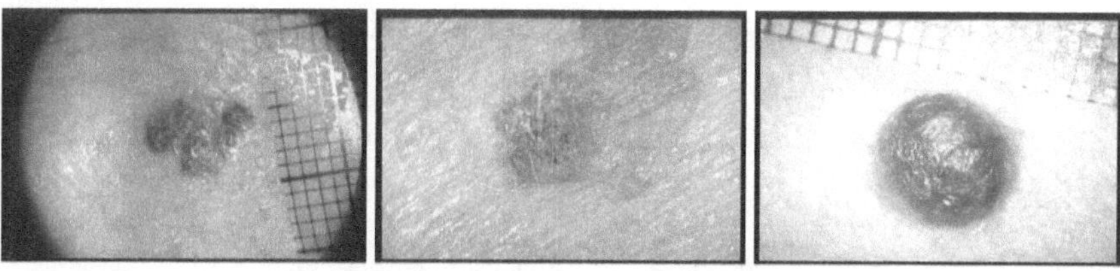

Figure 2.4: Examples of Seborrheic Keratosis [4]

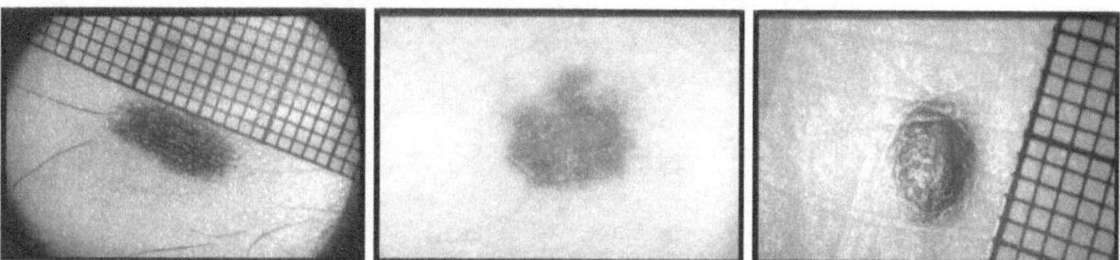

Figure 2.5: Examples of Nevus [4]

2.3.2 Screening for skin cancer

Screening is the process of performing a preemptive search for a cancer before a patient shows symptoms [67]. This results in the identification problem areas that are monitored by both the patients and doctors, quickly catching any lesion that becomes cancerous. There are attempts to implement general screenings for skin cancer however the process is not simple.

The complications arise from various factors. First there is the large variety of shapes, sizes, coloration, amongst others, that skin lesions can take. Many lesions are not malignant, even if they resemble a cancerous lesion, so a high degree of expertise is required to correctly classify a lesion. On top of that, previously benign lesions can mutate into cancer, so, even from the benign lesions, some have to be placed under surveillance. The fact that the whole perimeter of the body must be examined, coupled with some difficult decisions extends the time required to perform the screening task.

Screening for skin cancer entails the visual observing the skin in the search for nevi, or other pigmented areas that look abnormal in color, size, shape, or texture [67]. Other factors that increase the likelihood of skin cancer are also documented. Factors like sunburnt areas, especially those that are not recovering properly, fair skin, the patient using tanning beds, being older than 60 or having a weak immune system all contribute to a higher chance of skin cancer occurring [8].

If not for the extremely varied nature of the cancerous lesions, the screening process could be performed by regular medical staff, with minimal training. Attempts have been done in order to streamline the classification of cancerous lesions. The identification of common irregularities lead to the introduction of several methods that can quantify the likelihood of a lesion being cancerous.

These methods improved the diagnostic performance of less experienced dermatologists. However they fail to address the reproducibility problem of the diagnosis, even amongst experts [52].

Teledermatology aids in the screening process, as the medical staff can be educated in what constitutes a dangerous lesion, leaving the precise classification for the expert. This method expands the number of medical staff that is now qualified to perform the screening process, making it a more viable solution as well as reducing wait times for when the procedure is utilized [47].

Identifying cancerous lesions early is critical to increase the survivability of the patient, however this does not mean that the screening process is a perfect solution without drawbacks.

2.3.3 Drawbacks of screening for skin cancer

Before stating the drawbacks, it is note worthy to point out that, in addition to increasing the survivability of the patient, documenting dangerous lesions that later become cancerous provides useful data for future screenings, diagnosis and construction of automatic classifiers.

Although largely beneficial, screening has valid problems. These mainly originate from the lack of a simple and accurate diagnosis method [8, 67]. First, the screening process itself takes a considerable amount of time to be conducted, as the whole body needs to be observed. Skin cancer is more likely to develop in sun-exposed areas, but it can also occur in protected/hidden areas such as the genitalia.

Due to the complicated nature of the lesions, their large variations in shape, color and texture, they require the opinions of an expert for classification. However, obtaining the opinion of an expert takes too much time due to the inadequate number of professionals [32] and the large gap in experience [35] each expert can have.

Incorrect classification of a lesion carries problems independent of screening. However screening increases the number of lesions that are classified, leading to eventual incorrect classifications. This is a problem in screening as, in the large majority of the time, the classified skin lesions have shown no symptoms or other evidence to suggest the need for medical care. From a misclassification, two outcomes can occur. If a cancer is incorrectly classified as benign, the malignant lesion is given more time to progress, with the possibility of the patient delaying getting medical care despite having symptoms. If a benign lesion is misclassified as cancerous, the patient could suffer from anxiety, as well as receiving further treatment that would be costly and have side effects. There is also the possibility of leaving permanent damage such as scars from the excision of the lesion [67].

Lastly, the method generally used to diagnose the cancer is the biopsy. This operation requires the extraction of the lesion, either in its entirety or only portions, so that it can then be analysed by a pathologist. The operation is invasive, with the possibility of causing infection and scarring [67].

An important note is the existence of studies that show that screening for skin cancer has not led to a decrease in the chances of dying from skin cancer [67].

These set of factors have led to some organizations not having an opinion on whether to recommend or oppose the promotion of the screening of skin cancer [8]

With the recent developments of various technologies, various machine learning algorithms started to produce better results in this area. Although these algorithms will not replace the experts, they can be used to provide a reliable second opinion on a lesion.

2.4   Skin cancer data sets

Skin cancer cases have been documented in the medical record of the patients with the format of pictures and description/annotation of important structures. The datasets are made from these medical records and have some common problems. The data in the medical record of patients is confidential, so access to it is complicated. Each hospital/clinic/university hospital has different formats for their medical records, as well as the data (images), being acquired with different equipment and techniques (the images were acquired with different cameras and conditions). As such, the samples from a dataset may vary considerable from samples of another dataset, making it difficult to compare the obtained results.

Another problem is that different datasets were created with different objectives in mind. Some are created with a focus on separating Nevus from Melanoma, others to differentiate cancer from non-cancer (involving various types of skin cancer, not just Melanoma (MEL)). As such the number of classes or data types for each datasets can vary, making it more difficult to join them together without loosing information.

A big problem with the datasets from this domain is their low availability, coupled with the low number of samples. Although recently there has been an effort to congregate large numbers of samples and making them public [40], the majority of the datasets in the literature are private. Even those that are public contain a small number of samples. Some authors complimented public datasets with their privately obtained datasets. Be it due to the low number of samples from the public datasets, or intending to increase the diversity of their data, in the end the larger datasets were never released to the public.

A total of 24 datasets were considered. They are here described with as much information as was made available. For brevity, the classes that each dataset contains (when stated) are abbreviated, with only the classes that are used in this work specifically specified.

The datasets of DermIS [23], Dermnet [22] and Dermnet NZ [69] were obtained from online archives. These online archives contain a large amount of data within, however this data is spread across many specific skin cancers, with some containing only a few (1 2) samples. The data is publicly available, however contains a watermark. The original, higher quality, data can usually be obtained by requesting it from the website owners, or by paying a fee.

DermIS [23] originates from the University of Heidelburg and Erlangen, Germany. The largest reported usage mentions 397 clinical images and metadata, including melanoma and nevi skin lesions. The images have been reported to have varying resolutions (from 550×367 to 550×469) and hair. Dermnet [22] contains around 23,000 images, as of 2016, while DermNet NZ [69] contains more than 25,000 clinical or dermoscopy images, as of 2020. Their resolutions and quality vary from image to image.

DermQuest [29] would be another online medical archive but ended up losing support and being discontinued in 2019/12/31, however most of their database can be found in the SD-198 [78] dataset. The SD-198 is a dataset made from data available on the DermQuest site at the time of its creation on 2016. It contains a total of 6,584 images from 198 classes, these include different diseases from different types of eczema, acne and various cancerous conditions as well as lesions in hard-to-diagnose places.

Two of the datasets were obtained from Dermoscopy Atlases. The datasets are the Sydney Melanoma Diagnostic Centre at the Royal Prince Alfred Hospital [57] and the Interactive atlas of Dermoscopy: A tutorial (also known as EDRA) made by Argenziano et al. [4] from the university hospital of Graz, Austria, university hospital of Naples, Italy, and university hospital of Florence, Italy. Their images are true color, have a resolution of 768×512 pixels, have similar quality and some samples contained lesions that exceeded the border of the image. The first Atlas contains 168 clinical images, divided into benign and melanoma classes. The second Atlas contained 1011 lesions with clinical image, dermoscopic image, metadata and the 7-point classification for each sample. the dataset is divided into 20 classes, with the more prominent classes being BCC, Nevus, Miscellaneous (MISC), SK and MEL. Although both started as private, the Interactive atlas of Dermoscopy: A tutorial [4] was later released together with a study by Kawahara et al. [44].

The MED-NODE [31], PH2 [56], Dermofit [6], HAM10000 [81], BCN20000 [19] and ISIC archive [40] are datasets that are available to the public. Of these, only the Dermofit dataset has a one-off pay requirement. The MED-NODE [31] dataset was created with images from the Department of Dermatology of the University Medical Center Groningen, Netherlands. These images were acquired using a Nikon D3 or Nikon D1x body and a Nikkor 2.8/105 mm micro lens and lighting provided by two Multiblitz Variolite 600 flash units with a color temperature equal to 5200 Kelvin. A total of 170 clinical images, divided into MEL and NEV, was selected from the hospital. The images were manually processed to remove distracting elements, like clothes, and obtrusions, like hairs, ensuring the focus of the images were the lesion and some surrounding healthy skin.

The PH2 [56] dataset was made in a joint research collaboration between the Universidade do Porto, Técnico Lisboa, and the Dermatology service of Hospital Pedro Hispano in Matosinhos, Portugal. The images are obtained under the same conditions through Tuebinger Mole Analyzer system with a magnification of $20\times$, resulting in 8-bit RGB color images with a resolution of 768×560 pixels resolution. A total of 200 dermoscopic images and metadata, divided into NEV and MEL, were chosen with the best quality, resolution and features. The metadata includes observed criteria from the lesions that is considered informative to the diagnosis, these being majorly features required for methods such as the ABCD rule, 7-point method and Menzies method.

The Dermofit dataset [6] was compiled from the University of Edinburgh, Scotland, consisting of 1300 focal high quality clinical images, and their segmentation mask, divided into 10 classes. The more recognisable classes are the BCC, NEV, SK, Squamous Cell Carcinoma and MEL. The images were acquired with a Canon EOS 350D SLR camera, with the lighting being controlled using a ring flash and all images captured at the same distance (50 cm) resulting in a pixel resolution of about 0.03 mm.

The Ham10000 [81] contains a total of 10015 dermoscopic images and metadata, divided into 7 classes. The more recognisable classes are the BCC, NEV and MEL. The images were acquired from the Department of Dermatology at the Medical University of Vienna, Austria, and the skin cancer practice of Cliff Rosendahl in Queensland, Australia.

The BCN20000 [19] contains 19424 dermoscopic high-quality images and metadata from 5583 skin lesions, divided into 8 classes. The more recognisable classes are the BCC, NEV, SK, Squamous Cell Carcinoma and MEL. The images were obtained from the Hospital Clínic de Barcelona, Spain. The acquisition was done by a set of dermoscopic attachments on three high-resolution cameras with the images being pre-processed by several computer vision algorithms.

The ISIC archive [40], is a compilation of several datasets (various clinics, MSK (IE ISIC2017) [17], HAM10000 [81] and BCN20000 [19]), both public and private, managed by the International Skin Imaging Collaboration (ISIC), an academia and industry partnership designed to facilitate the application of digital skin imaging to help reduce melanoma mortality. The ISIC organization as been launching yearly competitions since 2016, creating the yearly ISIC datasets, with the purpose of furthering the technology related to Computer-Aided Diagnosis (CAD) systems. The ISIC [year] datasets are then integrated into the ISIC archive [40] and made public. The ISIC organization maintains a set standard of quality and method that they enforce on all data that they include in their database.

ISIC 2016 [34] is the first challenge launched by the ISIC organization, the dataset contained a total of 1250 images with a hand-made segmentation mask and metadata. Only two classes were considered, either Malignant of Benign.

ISIC 2017 [17] dataset contained a total of 2750 images and metadata, pre-partitioned into training, validation and testing portions. The images were obtained from leading clinical centers internationally and acquired from a variety of devices within each center. Three classes were considered, MEL, NEV or SK.

ISIC 2018 [16], in this challenge the dataset of the HAM10000 [81] was included, among others, resulting in a total of 11720 images. The images from HAM10000 were used as training data while the remaining images were used for validation or testing. A total of 7 classes were considered, with the more recognisable classes are the BCC, NEV and MEL.

ISIC 2019 [41] dataset included the previous two challenges datasets, as well as a new one, the BCN20000 [19], totaling in around 33894 images. A total of 9 classes were considered. The more recognisable classes are BCC, NEV and MEL.

Several authors utilized images from private sources in addition to public sources, not releasing their datasets. Shimizu et al. [75] added samples from the Keio University Hospital and Tokyo Women's Medical University, Japan to the EDRA dataset [4]. In total, 964 dermoscopy images were used, divided into MEL, NEV, BCC and SK. The images had differing resolutions, ranging from 512×384 to 3641×2732.

Esteva et al. [24] joined samples from the Stanford Hospital, California, USA, with plublic datasets from the ISIC Archive [40] and the Dermofit library [6]. This dataset contained a total of 129,405 images, divided into benign lesions, malignant lesions and non-neoplastic lesions. Images that were blurry, far from the lesion or were from the same lesion (different points of view) were limited to the training set of the dataset.

Haenssle et al. [35] joined 300 high-quality images, divided into MEL and NEV, from the University of Heidelberg and with the dataset from the ISIC 2016 challenge [34]. The images were obtained with a variety of combinations of cameras and dermatoscopes.

Kharazmi et al. [46] joined samples from the University of Missouri, USA and Vancouver Skin Care Centre, Canada, with the EDRA [4] dataset. This dataset contained a total of 1199 RGB dermoscopy images and metadata, divided into BCC and non-BCC classes. The quality of the images and camera utilized is not mentioned for the University of Missouri, USA, while the Vancouver Skin Care Centre, Canada utilized a Dermlite smartphone dermoscope with polarized light, ie, "dry" dermoscopy.

Other utilized solely private datasets like Fujisawa et al. [28] that utilized samples from the University of Tsukuba Hospital, Japan. This dataset contained 6009 images, divided into 21 specific classes. Of these, the Squamous Cell Carcinoma, BCC, MEL, SK, NEV and MISC are the more recognisable. The images were taken with a digital cameras with at least 6 million pixels, macro lens, macro ring flash, at various distances and from different angles, with some lesions having been photographed multiple times, such as in close-up or at different angles when the tumour was protruding from the surface.

Tschandl et al. [82] utilized samples from the primary skin cancer clinic in Queensland, Australia. This dataset contained 14699 images, 6464 clinical and 8235 dermoscopic images, divided into 10 classes. Of these, the BCC, MEL, NEV and Squamous Cell Carcinoma are the more recognisable. The images were obtained with different cameras, dermatoscopes, resolutions and with polarizing mode either on or off. In addition, close-up images were taken with a spacer attached to the digital single-lens reflex camera, removing all incident light and standardizing distance and field of view.

Ly et al. [50] compiled several publicly available datasets into the PHDB dataset, but did not release it to the public. This dataset was made from the ISIC Archive [40], Dermnet NZ [69],

MED-NODE [31] and PH2 [56].

Lastly, the quality of the images in the datasets is often incomplete or not described at all. However, from those that describe it, and our personal experience, the images usually face problems with the skin hair, contrast between lesion and background skin, identifiable body parts(nose), uneven illumination or air bubbles [48]. Even when the quality of the images is stated to be high, some images contain one or more of the above problems.

The above datasets are summarized relative to their release date, name, type of data included, number of samples and accessibility in Table 2.1. An observation is that the number of samples increase with the passing of the years, however a large leap is made around 2016, were datasets containing more than 10,000 samples are used. Although the table shows a large number of public datasets a careful observation will reveal that half of the public datasets are included in other public datasets. This is the case for the yearly ISIC datasets, as well as the HAM10000 and BCN20000, that can be included in the ISIC Archive. Other public datasets, such as the DermIS, Demnet, Dermnet NZ and Dermofit have either to be requested, or paid for, but are other wise available. The SD-198 dataset is available, however the way to obtain it has been lost. The Samples column indicates the number of samples used in the literature, as such, some public datasets have a "NA" in the number of samples as they either have not been used, or can not be separated from other datasets in the literature.

Table 2.1: List of encountered datasets, their date, data type, samples and their accessibility.

Date	[REF] Dataset	Data Type	Samples	Accessibility
2010	[23] DermIS	clinical metadata	397	public
1998 2016	[22] Dermnet	clinical	NA	public
1996 2020	[69] Dermnet NZ	clinical	NA	public
2019	[29] DermQuest	NA	NA	deactivated
2016	[78] SD-198	clinical	6,584	NA
2003	[57] Sydney Melanoma Diagnostic Centre at Royal Prince Alfred Hospital	clinical	168	private
2002	[4] EDRA	clinical dermoscopic metadata	1011	public
2015	[31] MED-NODE	clinical	170	public
2013	[56] PH2	dermoscopic metadata	200	public
2008 2017	[6] Dermofit	clinical	1300	public

Date	[REF] Dataset	Data Type	Samples	Accessibility
2018	[81] HAM10000	dermoscopic metadata	10015	public
2019	[19] BCN20000	dermoscopic metadata	19424	public
2016 2019	[40] ISIC Archive	clinical dermoscopic metadata	NA	public
2016	[34] ISIC 2016	dermoscopic metadata	1250	public
2017	[17] ISIC 2017	dermoscopic metadata	2750	public
2018	[16] ISIC 2018	dermoscopic metadata	11720	public
2019	[41] ISIC 2019	dermoscopic metadata	33894	public
2015	[75] Keio University Hospital, Japan Tokyo Women's Medical University, Japan	dermoscopic	645	private
2017	[24] Stanford Hospital	dermoscopic	NA	public
2018	[35] University of Heidelberg, Germany	clinical dermoscopic	300	private
2018	[46] The University of Missouri, USA Vancouver Skin Care Centre, Canada	dermoscopic metadata	1199	private
2003 2016	[28] University of Tsukuba Hospital	clinical	6009	private
2008 2017	[82] Primary skin cancer clinic in Queensland, Australia	clinical dermoscopic	14699	private
2018	[50] PHDB	dermoscopic metadata	NA	private
End of table				

From these datasets, only those that are publicly available can be used. This work requires that the dataset needs to have at least both image types and metadata. Of the 24 above described datasets, only the ISIC Archive and EDRA meets the requirements. Finally the EDRA dataset is adopted as its use in an interesting paper by Kawahara et al. [44], where a multimodal and multitasking approach is investigated, can be replicated, making comparisons with said paper more reliable.

Chapter 3

Literature review

With the improvements in the digitalisation of the samples, new opportunities for the field of image processing and bioinformatics have appeared. This, coupled with the inadequate number of dermatologists [32] and the growing number of cancerous lesions, raised a lot of interest, with a considerable number of researchers conducting a large amount of work related to the development of a Computer-Aided Diagnosis (CAD) system.

The background for machine learning, an introduction, the classifiers, deep learning and evaluation is presented in Section 3.1. An overview of the CAD systems is shown in Section 3.2. After an introduction and explanation of CAD systems, the various pre-processing and augmentation techniques utilized are summarized in Sub-Section 3.2.1. Segmentation is explained in Section 3.2.2, together with the methods utilized to perform it. Features extracted and the selection methods are shown in Sub-Section 3.2.3. The classifiers utilized are demonstrated in Sub-Section 3.2.4. Multimodal CAD systems are further explored in Sub-Section 3.2.5 before a summary of the conclusions obtained from the literature is presented in Section 3.3.

3.1 Background on machine learning

Machine learning is the creation of a "machine" by a learning algorithm that can solve the desired problem with the available data. This method is an alternate solution to those obtained through conventional engineering. While to engineer a conventional solution, the domain knowledge needs to be extracted from the problem and then an optimized algorithm can be built to suit the problem. Machine learning does not require the discovery of the domain knowledge, or the hand crafting of an algorithm. Rather, a sufficiently large number of examples are utilized by the learning algorithm to produce a model for the examples. With this model, other examples can be fitted in a pattern [76]. Due to this, machine learning can more easily provide answers to complex problems, without requiring too much specific knowledge on the problem.

The disadvantage is that the quality of the machine learning solution is not guaranteed, as its performance is based on the domain knowledge obtained from the previous examples, as well as not being optimized for the problem.

In the machine learning field, three types of learning can happen depending on the task intended to perform. When the task is that of matching data to a desired label, supervised learning is being performed. This type of learning is common to be applied when the data is labeled, intending to match the input data with the desired output label. When the task is identifying/discovering common characteristics between the data, unsupervised learning is being performed. Applied in occasions where new knowledge of the data is desired, unsupervised learning discovers common characteristics between the data to group it accordingly, finding useful connections that might have gone unnoticed. When the task is to learn in an interactive environment, reinforcement learning is being performed. In it, the feedback from interacting with the environment through trial and error is used to guide the learning.

When supervised and unsupervised learning are applied to continuous and discrete data, it can be further sub classified. Supervised learning task can be regression (label is numeric) or classification (label is categorical). Unsupervised learning falls usually into two categories: clustering and association rules.

Given the objective to link a given set of input data (images and/or metadata) into one of various possible categorical labels (skin cancers), the learning task performed is that of supervised learning, namely the classification. Several learning algorithms can be used within this particular learning task. These algorithms that implement classification, especially in a concrete implementation, are known as classifiers.

3.1.1 Classifiers

Several classifiers have been tried in the literature to perform skin cancer classification. Each classifier utilizes a different approach to create a machine capable of solving the problem. A short description for the classifiers utilized in the literature is shown here.

3.1.1.1 Naive Bayes

Naive Bayes assumes the independence between features, therefore computing a probability for each category for the given data [9].

3.1.1.2 Support Vector Machines

Support Vector Machines classifier, see in Figure 3.1, finds the optimal separating line that correctly classifies the data into their correct classes [9].

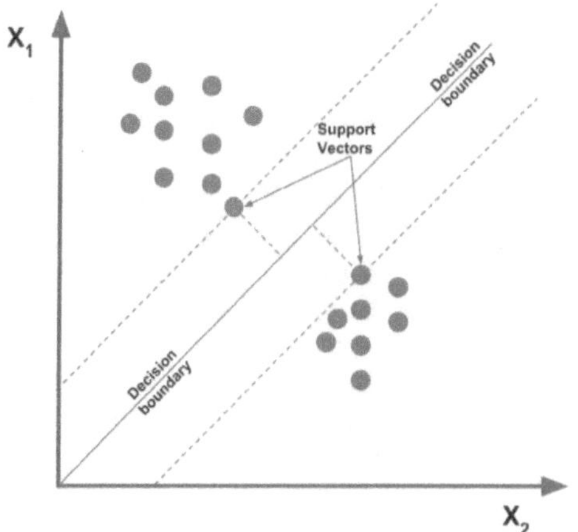

Figure 3.1: Example of a Support Vector Machine classifier, a decision boundary is identified that separates the data into the correct classes, with the data points that defined the decision boundary being the support vectors. Retrieved from [73].

3.1.1.3   K-Nearest Neighbors

The K-Nearest Neighbors classifier, seen in Figure 3.2, is the first of many non-linear classifiers, in it a distance function is used to determine the distance of each data sample from each other, a new sample is classified by its k nearest samples [9]. On the other hand, K-means projects the samples to a plane, where the samples are then divided into k clusters, each group having a calculated centroid, with new samples being classified according to their distance from the centroids [9].

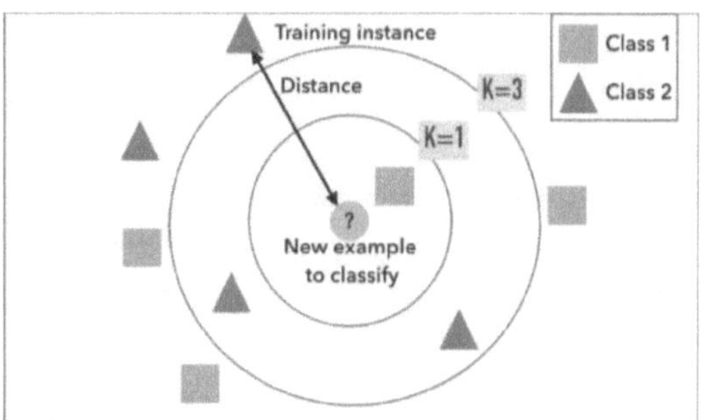

Figure 3.2: Example of a K-Nearest Neighbors classifier. The distance from each data instance and the example is calculated, with the nearest K instances used to classify the new sample. K=1 would classify it as class 1, while K=3 would classify it as class 2. Retrieved from [77].

3.1.1.4 Decision trees

Decision trees, seen in Figure 3.3, are also utilised. These classifiers construct a decision process where each branch represents a good separation point between samples, where most of the samples of a class are isolated, the decision process ends in the leaves, that represent the target classes [3]. Random Forests extend on the decision trees classifier by utilizing several decision trees, each decision tree is exposed to different groupings of data with the objective of having the decision trees find and focus on an important aspect of the problem, culminating in a better result [36].

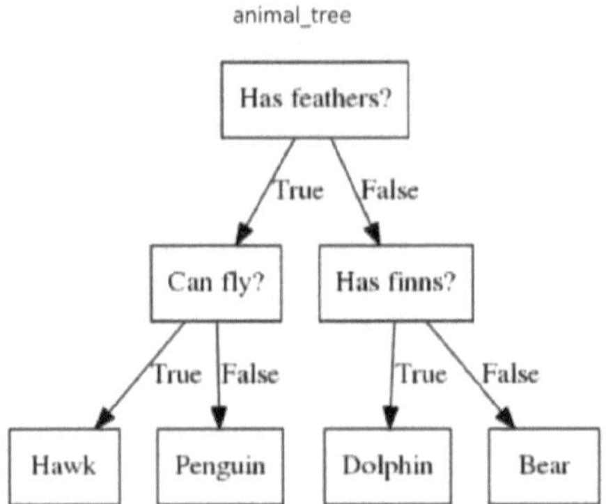

Figure 3.3: Example of a decision tree classifier. Questions about the data are used to divide the data until each class is clearly separated from each other, creating an easy to understand inquiry that leads to a correct classification of the data. Retrieved from [14].

3.1.1.5 Ensemble learning

Similar to random forests, ensemble learning, seen in Figure 3.4, consists of training several classifiers, with the prediction being based on the predictions from these. However, contrary to random forests, ensemble learning does not utilize only a type of classifier, this allows for the problem to be addressed with different approaches [70] as well as utilizing different systems to fuse the results, such as majority voting (where the prediction with the most classifiers wins). AdaBoost (short for Adaptive Boosting) extends on the ensemble technique by biasing some of the classifiers to handle outliers in the data [27].

3.1.2 Deep learning

By imitating the brain, Artificial Neural Network utilize nodes to copy the behaviour of

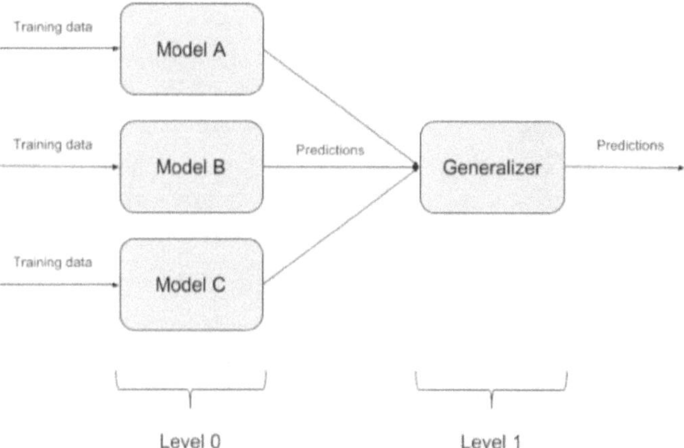

Figure 3.4: Example of ensemble learning. Several models are utilized to classify the data. The final classification is derived from generalizing the classifications from each model. Retrieved from [13]

neurons. The nodes are arranged in layers, with each node generally being connected to nodes in the previous and next layers. Data is introduced in the input layer where it then travels the length of the network, being changed by the nodes, until it arrives at the output layer and activates the appropriate nodes that indicate the classifiers prediction. The behaviour of the nodes is updated by a back propagation algorithm so that the prediction of the model matches the truth [33]. More specifically, it is the Deep Neural Network (DNN) branch of the Artificial Neural Network that is being utilized the most. DNN, seen in Figure 3.5, vary from the normal Neural Network (NN) by having a considerably larger number of layers [33]. This larger number of layers allows the network to extract better features from the data.

Convolutional Neural Network are a DNN that utilize Convolutional layers to extract features from images. The Convolutional layers generates abstract representations of the input image, from which features are extracted for classification. These abstractions are represented in the increase of the channels. Other layers that can occur are the Batch Normalization layer, the ReLU Non-linearity layer and the MaxPooling layer. The Batch Normalization layer normalizes the data by applying a transformation that maintains the mean output close to 0 and the output standard deviation close to 1. The ReLU Non-linearity layer applies the standard ReLU activation ($max(x, 0)$), avoiding the occurrence of negative values. The MaxPooling layers reduces the dimensionality of the data.

NN are easier to implement as they allow for a greater abstraction from the domain knowledge, however their operation after training is difficult to understand, leading to a difficulty in explaining the predictions. This problem is aggravated in DNN, as the largest difference is the number

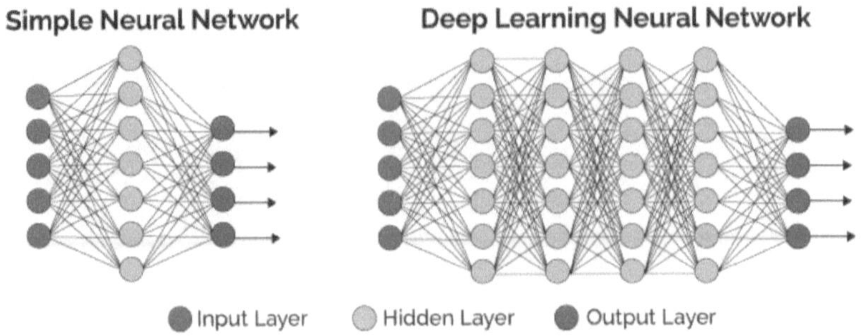

Figure 3.5: Example of a NN on the left and a DNN on the right. The Simple network on the left is made up of a single (to few) hidden layers, while the DNN on the right necessarily contains several hidden layers. Retrieved from [83].

of layers. The increase in the number of layers allows the network to extract better features, however the network requires additional data to improve. Another benefit of using DNN is the ability of using existing networks and the resources spent training them on other learning tasks with similar data formats. This is achieved by copying the network and using the Transfer learning technique. In it, the knowledge (weights and bias) of the existing network is transferred to the new network. The new network is then trained on the actual data to fine-tune it to the intended learning task.

3.1.3 Validation methods and evaluation

The models have to be validated to ensure that the results obtained are a reflection of the real-world scenario. Several methods to validate are available such as the Train/test split where data is randomly split into, usually, 70% for training and 30% for testing. k-Fold Cross-Validation divides the data into k folds of data. K models are trained, each having a different data fold used as the testing fold, with the others used as training. This validation method allows the whole dataset to be used to train the model, reducing the changes of the model missing a particular case that has few samples. Leave-one-out Cross-Validation takes the previous method to the extreme by training the model on all but one sample of the data [33]. Usually, a "validation set" is used to adjust parameters. In the Train/test split, this would be a subset of the training set, while with k-Fold Cross-Validation it would be internal cross-validation.

CAD systems are evaluated by the evaluation metrics. Due to the danger involved in this domain, no one metric is favoured above another, with different metrics evaluating the model from different perspectives. The evaluation metrics are calculated from the comparison of the predictions from the model with the true predictions.

The comparison can be projected to a confusion matrix. The confusion matrix is a two-dimensional matrix, one dimension contains the predicted label, while the other dimension contains the true label [80]. Generally it contains only positive and negative labels. When there are more than two possible labels, the matrix becomes a multilabel confusion matrix. Most of the other metrics are calculated from this matrix.

The accuracy metric indicates how close the results come to the truth. It is calculated by dividing the sum of true positives (correctly predicted malignant lesions) and true negatives (correctly predicted benign lesions) by the total number of samples. Achieving a high accuracy score is ideal, however, for this domain of skin cancer, when misclassifying a malignant lesion as benign (False Negative) is considerably more dangerous than the other way around, doctors prefer to take in consideration other metrics such as Sensitivity (SEN) or Specificity (SPC).

Sensitivity/True Positive Rate/Recall is a statistical measure that shows the proportion of true positives within the total of positive predictions (predicted malignant lesion), calculated following the equation in 3.1. While Specificity/Selectivity/True Negative Rate is a statistical measure that shows the proportion of true negatives within the total of negative predictions (predicted benign lesion), calculated following the equation in 3.2 [2]. In other words, SEN shows the probability of a positive prediction being correct while SPC shows the probability of a negative prediction being correct.

$$\frac{True positives}{True positives + False Negatives} \tag{3.1}$$

$$\frac{True Negatives}{True Negatives + False Positives} \tag{3.2}$$

The F1 score is another measure of accuracy. It focuses more on the positive predictions by being calculated from the precision metric (3.4) and the recall (or SEN) metric . It is calculated using the equation in 3.4.This indicates the harmonic mean of the precision and recall. The highest possible value is 1. Obtaining it indicates a perfect precision and recall, while a 0 is obtained if either precision or recall is 0.

$$\frac{\sum True positive}{\sum Predicted condition positive} \tag{3.3}$$

$$2 \times \frac{Precision \times Sensitivity}{Precision + Sensitivity} \tag{3.4}$$

Metrics such as the Receiver Operating Characteristic (ROC) curve and the accompanying Area under the receiver operating characteristic (AUROC) are also favoured by doctors. The ROC curve indicates the relationship between the true positive rate (TPR) and the false positive rate (FPR), while the AUROC estimates the discriminating power of the classifier. AUROC ranges from 0 to 1, with a perfect classifier obtaining a score of 1 and a score of 0.5 indicating the same discriminating power as randomly choosing the prediction [2].

3.2 Computer-Aided Diagnosis systems for skin cancer classification

CAD systems have been under investigation since 1987 [52], with various systems having been proposed in the literature.

Generally denominated as Computer-Aided Diagnosis systems, they are usually composed of 4 stages: Pre-processing, Segmentation, Feature extraction, and Classification [38]. First the data, commonly images, is pre-processed to be cleaned or artificially increased through data augmentation techniques. Afterwards, the images are segmented, a process were the area of the lesion is separated from the healthy skin. At this point features are extracted and selected to feed the classifier to produce a prediction.

The performance of the system is measured through various evaluation metrics calculated from the results. The metrics provide several points of view over the results from which the performance of the system can be evaluated.

Despite improving over the years, obtaining increased accuracy, sensitivity and specificity, there has not been a widespread adoption of CAD systems in the medical field due to a lack of trust. The systems are viewed as a black box [59], i.e. do not provide evidence for their classification, by the medical community, and have yet to go through a large scale clinical trial. This does not discourage researches, with there being a surge in the literature with CAD systems utilizing DNN to perform one or more of the stages. With their increased performance and abstraction from the domain, these methods are easier to utilize, when compared with more classical CAD systems, however the black box problem is aggravated as the workings of Artificial Neural Network are harder to understand in general than other methods. As such CAD systems can be divided in classical systems, Classical with Deep Learning (CDL), and deep learning only systems.

A CAD system is considered to belong to the classical group if it utilizes classical methods for all of the stages. A CAD system belongs in the CDL group if one or more DNNs is utilized to perform any of the stages. While a CAD system belongs to the deep learning only group if every stage is performed by a DNN. The division of the systems along these groupings can be observed in Table 3.1. The table shows the paper reference, if pre-processing was performed, stages that did not utilize deep learning (X), the datasets used, along with the obtained accuracy, sensitivity and specificity (if mentioned).

The pre-processing stage is the only stage that is independent, with all groups having systems with it and without it. Of the systems that fit in the CDL group, see Table 3.1, all utilize a DNN to perform the feature extraction, with the system in [72] choosing to perform feature selection with another method. Segmentation is the next stage to have a large portion of papers deciding to perform it with a DNN.

Table 3.1: Papers considered for this work, if they used pre-processing, their grouping according to the decision to not use a DNN component (X), the datasets utilized and the accuracy, sensitivity and specificity obtained (if available).

PR: utilized data from private datasets.

PP: Pre-processing.

Se: Segmentation

ES: Feature extraction and selection

Cl: Classifier

Paper	Year	PP	Se	ES	Cl	Dataset	ACC	SEN	SPC
Classical									
[66]	2010	Y	X	X	X	DermIS, Dermnet	88.41	88.31	88.53
[53]	2014	Y	X	X	X	PR	90	91	89
[74]	2014	Y	X	X	X	EDRA, PR	93.83	93.76	93.84
[45]	2019	Y	X	X	X	DermIS	96	97	96
[31]	2015	Y	X	X	X	MED-NODE	81	81	80
[7]	2015	N	X	X	X	PH2, EDRA		98	90
[79]	2014	Y	X	X	X	PR	87.1	86.4	88.1
[25]	2016	Y	X	X	X	PH2, DermIS, DermQuest	80	73.33	86.66
[6]	2013	Y	X	X	X	DERMOFIT	93.9		
[75]	2015	Y	X	X	X	EDRA, PR			
Classical with deep leaning									
[15]	2015	N			X	ISIC	93.1	94.9	92.8
[60]	2016	Y	X			MED-NODE	81	81	80
[43]	2016	Y	X			ISIC (2016)	70		
[72]	2019	Y		X	X	PH2, ISIC (2016, 2017)	94.8	94.5	98
[51]	2019	Y			X	ISIC (2016, 2017)	87.7		
Deep learning only									
[71]	2017	Y				ISIC	78.66	78.66	79.74
[24]	2017	N				ISIC, PR	72.1		
[35]	2018	N				ISIC, PR			
[28]	2019	Y				PR	92.4	96.3	89.5
[82]	2019	Y				PR			
[50]	2018	Y				ISIC, Dermnet NZ, MED-NODE, PH2		88.23	83.82
[46]	2018	N				EDRA, PR	91.1	85.3	94
[85]	2018	N				PR			
[44]	2019	N				EDRA	74.2	60.4	91.0

3.2.1 Pre-processing

In the Pre-processing stage, the data is processed to be cleaned, filtered and organized. Although predominant in classical systems, this stage is also performed in the other groups. Since the critical portion of the data is in the format of images, Pre-processing refers primarily to smoothing, applying color transformations [74], removing artifacts and to improve the lighting of the images [60]. Pre-processing makes the images generally clearer so that the features obtained are of a higher quality. Several algorithms and/or methods are utilised to clean the images. These included an algorithm based on adaptive modification of wavelet coefficients [66], gaussian smoothing [31], gaussian kernel [43], the application of one or several filters [53, 72, 79] such as a median filter, the identification and discarding of images that were not possible to clean [31, 43] and even the application of image cleaning software such as the "dull razor software" [25, 31]. There are works that do not clean their images [15, 24, 28, 35, 44, 46, 50, 82, 85] as the technology used in the acquisition or processing of the images, either already includes such cleaning processes or are powerful enough that the results do not change much with the exclusion of this stage. The majority of these works fall under the group of deep learning only systems.

Another development tied to the introduction of deep learning is data augmentation. Data augmentation is the increase of the amount of data by adding slightly modified copies of already existing data. This is done as the size of the dataset has a large impact on the performance of deep learning, however, the currently publicly available datasets are of a small size. The most common image augmentation technique is that of rotating the images to various angles [28, 50, 71, 72], however re-scaling, horizontal/vertical shifting or flipping, zooming and sheering [71, 82] are also utilized in some papers.

3.2.2 Segmentation

In the Segmentation stage, the region of the images that contains the lesion and the regions that contain surrounding healthy skin are identified and separated. Although usually performed by an algorithm, some works performed this stage manually [7] as their interest lied in the feature extraction and classification stages. Others utilized statistical algorithms, like a histogram analysis based on fuzzy C-means [53] or statistical model based [6]. Another common algorithm utilized is the k-means [31, 45, 60, 79]. Others relied on more complex algorithms. Such as the snake segmentation technique [66], that allows for the stating of a starting delimitation, JSEG image segmentation algorithm [74], OpenCV's Canny edge detector [43] and even the combination of active contour with watershed algorithms [25].

DNN also perform well in this task. An example is a work that utilizes a sparse autoencoder [46] and another that utilizes two methods at the same time, a Convolutional Neural Network (CNN) (Caffe architecture) and a Sparse Coding SPAMS dictionary [15]. The remaining works all utilised DNN such as the VGG-19 [72], VGG-net [71], Google Inception v3 [24, 44], Google Inception v4 [35], GoogLeNet [28], ResNet-50 [85]. Some works even performed an ensemble of DNN, (AlexNet, VGGNet, ResNet-18 and ResNet-101) [51] and (inception V3 and ResNet50) [82].

There are multiple reasons for choosing to use a DNN over other, more conventional, methods. One such reason is the ability of using advanced and known networks, that have been proven to excel in a task similar to this one (image recognition). Another is the ability to transfer the knowledge obtained by those networks, acquiring a capable algorithm that takes little time to tune to the new domain. However, the work performed in [50] shows that DNN are not dependent on these advantages to achieve the same or higher performances. One problem that comes from utilizing these DNN, is their requirement of large amounts of data (images and their masks) to train these networks. Although an increasing number of larger datasets have been made public, it remains difficult to find datasets with both images and their masks.

3.2.3   Feature extraction and selection

In the Feature extraction and selection stage features are extracted from the data, with the best features being found and selected to be used by the classifiers to produce a prediction. Features are descriptions of the data that are understood by the classifiers. While some modalities, like metadata, can be directly translated as features, others, like images, require a complex process to be translated into meaningful features.

Features extracted from images are generally based on shape, color and texture of the lesion. Classical systems employed a variety of algorithms and methods to extract meaningful features. Shape features are among the more difficult to acquire, with only a minority of works obtaining them. These are generally the asymmetry [25, 66, 74], irregularity [66], size [25, 74], compactness [25, 74], ulnar variance [25], aspect ratio [74], eccentricity [74] and solidity [74] of the lesion. Although difficult to obtain, one could argue that the shape features are important, as a good portion of these are the criteria analysed within the ABCD rule. Asymmetry for A (Asymmetry), irregularity for B (Border irregularity) and size for D (Diameter larger than 6mm). Color is the only criteria that all of the works obtain features for.

Color features are usually statistical in nature and usually acquired from several different color spaces. The features are usually represented by the mean color [6, 31, 74], covariance matrices [6], an ad hoc color ratio [6], variance [25, 74, 79], standard deviation [31, 74, 75], minimum [75], maximum [75], average [75], skewness [25, 75] and entropy [25].

Variations of the Co-occurrence matrices, such as generalized co-occurrence matrices [6] and Gray Level Co-occurrence Matrix [25, 45, 53, 74, 75], are utilized to extract statistical features from the texture of the image. There are other methods that also provide texture features such as Grey-Tone Difference Matrix, Fuzzy-Mutual Information Based Wavelet Packet Transform and Autoregressive Modeling [53], as well as wavelet transformations and curvelet transformations [79].

The size of the lesion would be an excellent set of features to be extracted, however features related to the size of the lesion are hard to translate from images. This is due to there being no point of reference, or the methods used to extract features not being able to translate this information from the image. This does not discourage the attempt at calculating the size of the lesion, with several works implementing size equations that derive the size or diameter from other features [6, 25, 74]. However the majority of the works do not attempt to translate this set of features.

More recent works started to extract features from other regions of the lesion, dividing the features obtained into global and local features [7, 45, 75]. Global features represent an overview of the lesion, while local features represent the overview of important regions of the lesion such as the border, healthy skin, the lesion itself, and the combination of the lesion with the border. This approach attempts to copy the different aspects that a dermatologist can extract by comparing the features of each region to each other.

Many of the above mentioned methods and algorithms produce a large number of features, these however are not all necessarily meaningful to the prediction of the classifier. Passing all of the features to the classifier would muddy the prediction made, resulting in a poorer performance. Although some do not perform feature selection [15, 31, 53], selecting the best features should be done. Several methods are utilized throughout these works. A minority of them manually removed the under performing features [25], while the remaining used more automated methods. There are examples of the usage of the Principal Component Analysis [79], Wilks' Lambda step wise feature selection method [75] and a fast correlation-based feature filter [74]. A work tested several configurations of the Fisher's Linear Discriminant Analysis and Multiple Discriminant Analysis based on the Fukunaga-Koontz Transformation [66], with the second method performing the best.

Both of the groups of works with deep learning, CDL and deep learning only, preferred to leave both tasks, the extraction and selection, to the DNN [24, 28, 35, 44, 46, 50, 51, 60, 71, 82, 85]. Only two works deviated from this. In [72] a clustering controlled entropy method performed the feature selection. While in [15], in addition to the CNN, a Sparse Coding SPAMS dictionary is also used to obtain more features, with feature selection not being performed.

3.2.4   Classifiers

In the classification stage the selected features are fed to a classifier that produces a prediction on which type the lesion belongs to.

Many classifiers, and variations of, have been used in this stage for the systems. Their utilization itself is varied, with some works using a different classifier for each type of features [31] or overlapping various classifiers to produce two connected predictions [6].

The classifiers utilized include the Naive Bayes [66], Bayesian classifier [45], SVM (and derivatives) [7, 15, 25, 45, 53, 79], KNN [6, 7, 45], decision trees [45], AdaBoost [7], Random Forests [7], Artificial Neural Network [25, 72], CNN [60] and DNN [24, 28, 35, 43, 44, 46, 50, 51,

71, 82, 85].

Some works utilize an ensemble of classifiers. Several SVMs are trained on designed data subspaces, with the outputs merged using a NN in [74]. In [31], the color features are classified by a Cluster-based Adaptive Metric classifier, the texture features are classified by an Unbiased Color Image Analysis Learning Vector Quantization, metadata is classified with a naive Bayesian classifier, the final classification is done through majority voting. Another ensemble can be seen in [51], this time four different DNNs (AlexNet, VGGNet, ResNet-18 and ResNet-101) are utilized, with the fusion being done with an SVM classifier. In [6] a hierarchical K-Nearest Neighbors is utilized. Three KNNs are needed to establish the hierarchy, with the fist KNN differentiating from cancerous lesions and benign lesions and the last two further differentiating into a specific lesion classification.

3.2.5   Multimodality

Of the mentioned papers (Table 3.1), only five take advantage of the multiple modalities available to the domain. The majority of the works presented focus on a single image for each lesion, with two using images and metadata [31, 46], one using clinical and dermoscopic images [82], and two using clinical images, dermoscopic images and metadata [44, 85]. Considering the lack of multimodal research, this dissertation extends the state of the art in this area.

Giotis et al. [31] is the single paper from the classical group to utilize another modality. They obtained color and texture features from the images, these were each classified with their own classifier. The other modality was metadata, derived from the medical annotations on the lesion conforming to the lexicon of the PROVOKE system [30]. The metadata consisted of 10 categories, each with multiple possibilities. The categories encompassed the Part of the body, Spatial arrangement, Number of lesions, Size, 2-Dimensional shape, 3-Dimensional shape, Boundary sharpness, Color, Morphological group and texture of the surface. The metadata was classified as well with its own classifier, in this case a naive Bayesian classifier. The learning task was that of distinguishing melanoma lesions from benign nevi lesions. The metadata classifier obtained the best SEN at 0.78 (vs next 0.74) despite the lowest accuracy at 0.66 (vs next 0.73). The fusion of these classifiers was done through majority voting, obtaining 0.81 accuracy, 0.80 SEN and 0.81 SPC.

Kharazmi et al. [46] utilizes a Sparse Autoencoder to extract features from the image. These features are fused with metadata, being classified by a Softmax classifier. The metadata consists of 5 categories, Location, Size and Elevation of the lesion, as well as Age and Gender of the patient. The learning task is to separate Basal Cell Carcinoma (BCC) lesions from non-BCC lesions. Three results are shown, one using only the metadata, only the images and the final one where both modalities are fused. The metadata only results obtained a lower performance than image only, especially in the SEN (0.413 Meta-only vs 0.753 Img-only), while the results obtained from the usage of both modalities were the best at 0.911 accuracy, 0.853 SEN and 0.940 SPC. Despite a different learning task than [31], it can be observed a different result with the usage of metadata. This can be due to Giotis et al. utilizing more, and better, categories in the metadata than Kharazmi et al., however both obtain an improvement to the results by utilizing all of the modalities available.

The objective of Tschandl et al. [82] was to compare the accuracy of a CAD system utilizing deep learning to various medical personnel, with various levels of experience. The modalities consist of clinical images and dermoscopic images. Several DNNs were tested for each modality, with a ResNet50 architecture obtaining the highest accuracy with the clinical images, while an Inception V3 architecture obtained the highest accuracy with dermoscopic images. With the learning task of classifying the lesions into their precise classification, these were later grouped into cancerous and non-cancerous classifications. The model trained on the dermoscopic images obtained better results than the model trained on clinical images (0.725 vs 0.683 AUROC), however the fusion of both methods, utilizing extreme gradient boosting, obtained higher results with 0.74 AUROC, 0.81 SEN and 0.54 SPC.

Yap et al. [85] utilize clinical images, dermoscopic images and metadata to perform the classification of a lesion. Features from the images are extracted utilizing the ResNet50 architecture, with clinical images and dermoscopic images having their own ResNet50 feature extractor. The metadata consisted of 3 categories, age, gender and location of the lesion. The modalities are combined in a late fusion style by concatenating the features of the images with the metadata. The combined features are then forwarded through 2 fully connected layers before reaching the Softmax output layer. The best results were those of the clinical and dermoscopic combination and all data combination. The first achieved slightly higher AUROC for melanoma with results of 0.866 (vs 0.861), while the second achieved a slightly higher Mean average precision of 0.729 (vs 0.726). Both obtained the same AUROC for cancer (0.888). The metadata seems to have had an additional minimal impact on the results. With a more complex learning task and fewer categories in the metadata than Kharazmi this can indicate that the missing categories (size and elevation) are more important to the classification of a lesion. The other possibility is that the BCC cancer is more identifiable by the categories of the metadata.

Kawahara et al. [44] utilizes clinical images, dermoscopic images and metadata to perform multitasking. The learning tasks of skin lesion classification and 7-points categories classification are performed simultaneously in the same model. Features from the images are extracted utilizing an architecture from the ImageNet large scale visual recognition challenge, with clinical images and dermoscopic images having their own feature extractor. The metadata consisted of 3 categories, gender, location, and elevation of the lesion. In addition to several learning tasks being performed simultaneously, various combinations of modalities are proposed as well. These are performed in a late fusion fashion by concatenating the features of each modality (when needed). The combinations considered were those of dermoscopic images only; dermoscopic images and metadata; dermoscopic images, clinical images and metadata; clinical images and metadata; clinical images only. All of the learning tasks are repeated for each modality combination, with all combinations and all learning tasks being performed at the same time, in the same model. Classification is performed by a softmax classifier. The results for each combination are reported, with the accuracy of the lesion classification increasing in the order of clinical images; clinical images and metadata; dermoscopic images; dermoscopic images and metadata; and lastly the all-modalities combination, obtaining 74.2 accuracy, 60.4 average SEN, 91.0 average SPC and 0.896 average AUROC. Kawahara obtains a higher result compared to the work from Yap et al. [85] (0.896 vs 0.888 AUROC from Yap), however it is difficult to determine the factor behind this result. The classification of the categories of the 7-points in addition of the lesion classification, as well as the extra combinations preformed simultaneously are too large a difference in the methodology to ascribe to any of these as the principal responsible for the results. The fact remains that the results improved, even the inclusion of metadata improved the results, something that was ambiguous in Yap. The unambiguous improvement obtained by utilizing metadata can be due to Kawahara utilizing the elevation of the lesion, rather than age. Age is a much more broader descriptor for a lesion, and although an age over 50 is considered a risk factor for cancer [26], the elevation of the lesion is a more precise descriptor of the lesion in question.

3.3 Summary

Recent literature shows the usage of deep learning to be a good alternative for the more classical systems. Although the predictions are more difficult to explain, it requires less domain knowledge to be used. For this case, the knowledge required from image processing is reduced, as the features are automatically extracted by the network, rather than having to choose the features and designing a method to extract them. Works utilizing deep learning are obtaining results comparable to classical methods. These works are also able take advantage of developments from the area of image recognition, an area with high activity, as the networks utilized for in the CAD systems were first developed there. The literature mostly used proven architectures, with the advantage of transfer learning to boost the performance of the model. However these are large networks, needing a large amount of time to train, even when using transfer learning. As such, investigating the viability of a simpler architecture could be pursued. Due to the small size of the current publicly available datasets, data augmentation is required to increase the performance of deep learning.

Even dermatologists improve their diagnostic results when they have access to more data [35], however the number of studies that utilize more modalities is small compared the number of studies that utilize only one modality (images). Those that did saw that each modality obtained different results, but their combination acquired the best results.

The methods utilized in Kawahara et al. [44] brought an improvement to the results, in comparison to Yap et al. [85], however it is unclear which of the different methods utilized were responsible for this. Regardless, the multitasking performed in the work of Kawahara, the simultaneous performance of several learning tasks in the same model, seems a nice method to introduce additional data that is difficult to acquire. Data that would require analysis from a dermatologist, or other observations that are made at a later date, could be used to improve the performance of the model by being utilized as a learning task with multitasking. Another idea is to explore the effects of introducing the model to other modalities, such as metadata, with multitasking.

Transfer learning is regularly used to take advantage of experience from other similar domains, however it could be used to improve the training. Pre-training a model on a smaller set of modalities before transferring the knowledge to the model with all of the modalities could improve the performance of the model, or reduce the amount of training required.

Lastly, late fusion through concatenation of features and classification with a softmax classifier are the most common fusion technique and classifier used in the literature within the deep learning group.

Chapter 4

Experimental Methodology

In this chapter, the methodology used in this work to classify lesions is described. Since there are various modalities, the experiments focus around investigating their fusion with each other. The experiments range from a simpler, partial solution, utilizing unimodal data, to a mixture of data, to ending in a more complex solution that performs several fusions simultaneously. The experiments start with a baseline where a model is trained using only images and end in a model following the methodology proposed in [44].

Section 4.1 fully describes the dataset used in this dissertation. Section 4.2 explains the pre-processing steps related with data augmentation and balancing. Section 4.3 focus on the techniques used to build our deep neural network architectures: fusion, transfer learning and multitasking. Section 4.4 explains the building modules of the architectures used for training. Next, Section 4.5 presents the metrics used to assess the models and, finally, Section 4.6 describes each one of the experiments along with their objectives. A total of 11 experiments were developed, exploring multiple combinations of data, class and feature fusion, transfer learning and multitasking.

4.1 Dataset

The EDRA [4] dataset contains 1011 samples, each corresponding to different lesions. Each sample contains one clinical image, one dermoscopic image, metadata, the 7-point checklist, status for each of the 7-point checklist categories, and, lastly, the skin lesion classification. The metadata is made of three categorical variables. Elevation is the first, categorizing the elevation of a lesion as flat, palpable or nodular. The location indicates were the lesion is situated, possible being on the back, lower limbs, upper limbs, abdomen, chest, head neck, acral, buttocks or genital areas. Lastly there is the sex of the patient, either female or male.

Each sample has annotated the categories of the 7-point checklist. These categories track the existence and typicality of structures in the lesion that help distinguish it as malignant or benign. The categories of the 7-point checklist are: 1) Pigmented Network, which can be

Absent (ABS), Typical (TYP) or Atypical (ATP); 2) Blue Whitish Veil, ABS or Present (PRS); 3) Vascular modules, ABS, Regular (REG) or Irregular (IR); 4) Pigmentation, ABS, REG or IR; 5) Streaks, ABS, REG or IR; 6) Dots and Globules, ABS, REG or IR; And lastly, 7) Regression structures, either ABS or PRS. For cancer to be detected using the 7-point checklist, some of these categories must be present. Divided into 3 major and 4 minor categories, cancer is likely to be present if the summed score is equal or higher than 3. Any present criteria gives score, with minor criteria being worth 1 score, while the major are worth 2 score.

Lastly, there is the classification of the lesions/samples. The classifications are numerous and specific, however they were grouped following the same criteria as in [44] into Basal Cell Carcinoma (BCC), Nevus (NEV), Melanoma (MEL), Miscellaneous (MISC) or Seborrheic Keratosis (SK). The groupings can be seen in Table 4.1

Table 4.1: Full classifications and their groupings, adapted from [44].

Abreviation	Classification	# Images
BCC	basal cell carcinoma	42
NEV	blue nevus	28
	clark nevus	399
	combined nevus	13
	congenital nevus	17
	dermal nevus	17
	recurrent nevus	6
	reed or spitz nevus	79
MEL	melanoma	1
	melanoma (in situ)	64
	melanoma (less than 0.76 mm)	102
	melanoma (0.76 to 1.5 mm)	53
	melanoma (more than 1.5 mm)	28
	melanoma metastasis	4
MISC	dermatofibroma	20
	lentigo	24
	melanosis	16
	miscellaneous	8
	vascular lesion	29
SK	seborrheic keratosis	45

The categories of the 7-point checklist are distinct characteristics that can appear in a lesion, with these being important to the classification of a Melanoma. The focus of the work is the skin lesion classification. Since the 7-point checklist and lesion classification are correlated, this work also investigates the technique of multitask training by using as output the classification and the 7-point checklist categories.

One benefit of using this dataset is that it is publicly available, containing the split performed by Kawahara et al. in their work [44]. That way, our results can be directly compared with the results in the paper. The splits were adopted, splitting the 1011 samples into 413 train samples, 203 validation samples and 395 test samples (41/20/39% train/validation/test split).

As most real-world datasets in the health domain, classes are imbalanced. Figure 4.1 shows the distributions of the 5 types of lesion classification across the total, train, validation and test splits. NEV can be seen with the largest number of samples with 575 cases. MEL follows it with 252 cases, MISC with 97 cases, and the last two classes share the remaining 87 samples with BCC claiming 42 cases and SK with 45 cases. Despite this imbalance, the class distribution in the splits utilized by Kawahara et al. are proportional to the total of the dataset.

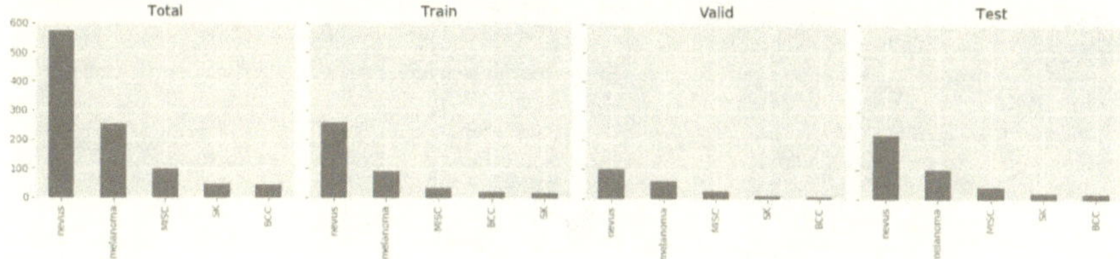

Figure 4.1: Distribution of the samples on the EDRA dataset.

Figure 4.2 shows examples from the EDRA dataset. Figures 4.2a and 4.2b are the clinical and dermoscopic images of a BCC lesion, while Figures 4.2c and 4.2d are the clinical and dermoscopic images of a MISC lesion. The images contain artifacts such as hair (4.2a and 4.2b), black border (4.2a and 4.2c) and objects like fingers (4.2c) and a black netting (4.2c and 4.2d). The dermoscopic images were captured with the usage of a dermatoscope. This device allows for more control over the environment and the acquisition of more details from the lesion. Dermoscopic images generally do not have light reflections or objects, with a special light being utilized to view modules in the inner layers of the skin. Clinical images, on the other hand, capture the lesion and some of its surrounding area, allowing for a better general view of the lesion and its shape.

4.2   Data pre-processing, augmentation and balancing

The images of the EDRA dataset are Red, Green and Blue (RGB) color images, with size of 768×512 pixels. The images were resized to 299×299 pixels with the nearest method to allow faster feature extraction. After resizing, the images were normalized, to the range of 0 to 1, by dividing by 255 so that the values of the images are better handled by the network, which is more suitable for the network architecture and parameters used.

The reduced number of samples and class imbalance is a problem in the dataset. A larger dataset would improve the performance of the model, while the imbalance of the classes introduces unwanted biases to the model. To address both problems, the need for more data and data balance,

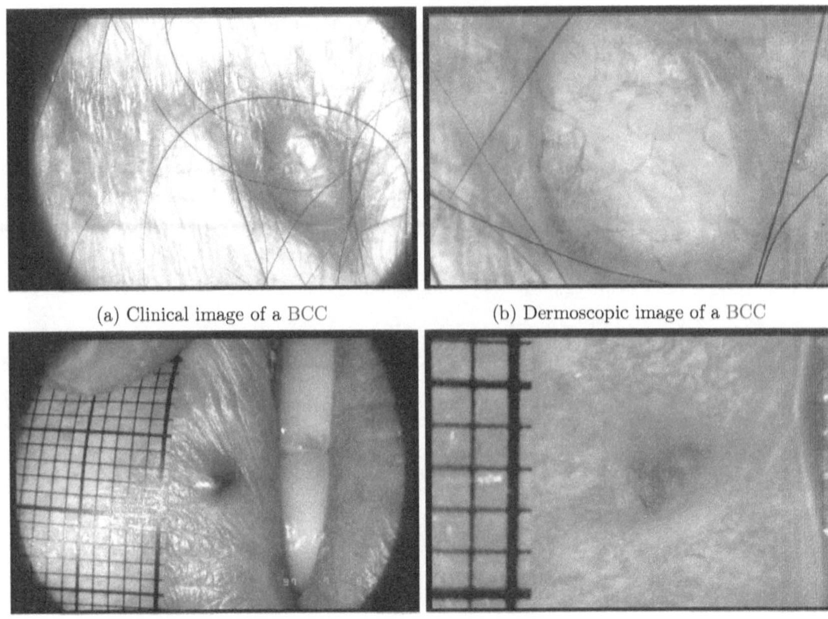

(a) Clinical image of a BCC   (b) Dermoscopic image of a BCC

(c) Clinical image of a MISC   (d) Dermoscopic image of a MISC

Figure 4.2: Example of clinical and dermoscopic images of a BCC lesion on the abdomen and a MISC lesion on the head neck.

data augmentation transformations were applied. To ensure reproducibility, a seed was used. The seed is a number used to start a pseudo-random number generator. The transformations to the images are then based on the numbers from the generator, which is started by the seed, ensuring that the augmentation was the same for the training of multiple models. Only the training split was augmented and balanced, as it is the data that will influence the model. The validation and testing splits were not augmented to make the results produced by these more comparable with other works performed on the dataset.

Several data augmentation transformations were applied:

- Horizontal flipping.

- Vertical flipping.

- Height shift with a maximum range of ten percent of the image size.

- Weight shift with a maximum range of ten percent of the image size.

- Rotations with a maximum range of $350°$ in both ways.

- Sheer with a maximum range of 0.15.

- Reflection filling mode, where blank space is filled with a reflection of the remaining image.

- Zoom range from 0.7% to 1.35%.

Examples of the transformations can be seen in Figure 4.7. Figure 4.3 is the original image. Figure 4.4 is the same image with transformations mainly regarding the flipping of the image, seen by the placement of the black grid, together with rotation and filling of the blank spaces, seen by the corners of the image. In Figure 4.5, flipping can be observed, together with zooming, seen in the increase in size of the lesion area (blue area). Lastly Figure 4.6 shows flipping, shifting, where the lesion area was moved (the top part of the image is cropped due to this), and a clearer vision of the filling mode, reflecting the final image on the blank space in the right side.

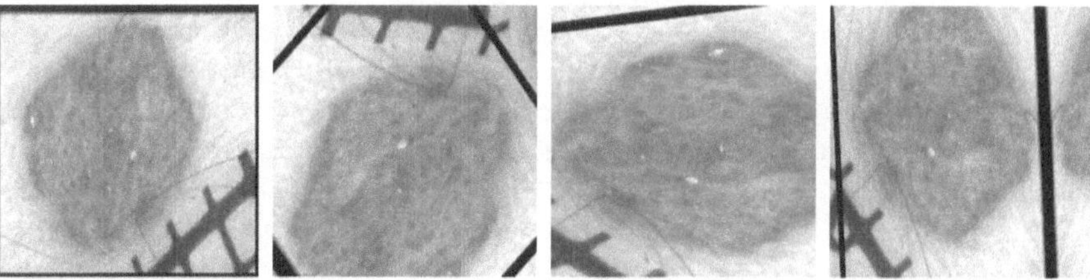

Figure 4.3: Original image   Figure 4.4: Flip and rotation   Figure 4.5: Flip and zoom   Figure 4.6: Flip, shift and reflection filling

Figure 4.7: Original image [5] and transformation examples derived from that image, each example is described with the most prevalent transformations.

By specifying so many aspects to be transformed, it is possible to create a large number of similar images. The pseudo-random number generator ensures that the created images do not follow a predictable pattern. As such, the created images are independent from the previous images. This independence and large number of possible images means that new images can be created as needed during the training of the model, removing the need to create a large database before the training. In total, around $18,500$ images were created for training, with $3,700$ images per class.

The performance of the skin lesion classification learning task is improved by using aditional tasks for learning (multitasking), namely the classification of the categories of the 7-point checklist. The skin lesion classification learning task is balanced with upsampling by augmentation, where the undersampled classes have more samples created. Upsampling by augmentation works with the skin lesion classification learning task, as it contains a small number of classes, results in a reasonable number of samples per class. However it is not suitable for multitasking classification, as by adding samples to a class from a particular learning task, it will also increase the number of samples for a different class of the other learning tasks. As such, the other learning tasks are balanced with a set of dynamic weights, updated every epoch.

4.3 Investigated techniques

Several techniques were examined to test their effects on the performances with respect to
the data and models used. First there is the data fusion techniques. In [7], it is shown that
late fusion provides better results compared with early fusion. As such, late fusion is explored
further, divided into class-fusion and feature-fusion. In class-fusion, each type of input data is
first classified independently. These classifications are then fused together by aggregation and
classified. In feature-fusion, features are extracted from each input data, fused by aggregation
and classified. Multitasking is used to perform several learning tasks at the same time. While
the skin lesion classification learning task is consistently performed, the other learning tasks,
when multitasking, are either the classification of the categories of the 7-point checklist or the
classification of metadata. Multitasking is used in this work as a way to bias the model towards
more meaningful features. The 7-point checklist is capable of determining if a lesion is cancerous
by focusing on 7 categories, while the metadata contains some information that is hard to acquire
(but useful) from the images. Transfer learning is utilized to transfer the weights and biases of
some experiments. This is done to investigate if the model performs better when parts of the
model are pre-trained on some modalities first, with multitasking the categories of the 7-point
checklist or the metadata.

4.4 Architecture

The classifier used is a small (low number of layers) Convolutional Neural Network (CNN),
inspired by the developments in the ISIC challenges [40] were more contestants have used CNN
approaches. The convolution layers utilized in these CNN have been proven to outperform
classical methods in analyzing images. The model built with the proposed network is able to
extract features from images, fuse multiple modalities, and classify the input data. The process
of extracting features from the images is integrated into the CNN as these networks are very
effective in extracting meaningfull information from the data, a necessity for handling high
dimensionality data such as images. The drawback of this choice is that it requires a large
amount of data, processing power, and a bigger network for the model to reach the reported
results in the literature. Time constraints and the large body of testing that is intended to be
performed favor the usage of a small network. This also serves to observe the behaviour of said
small network and its impact on the results.

To be able to perform these experiments, several modules pertaining to frequent operations
were created. Each experiment built its architecture utilizing only the modules it needed. The
initial architecture is a simple one, receiving only a single modality, a type of image, and the
output is the skin lesion classification. This simpler architecture serves to establish the backbone
of all of the following architectures, the feature extraction module. This module, seen in Figure 4.8,
is composed of an input layer, followed by four processing blocks. Each of the processing blocks
are made of a Convolutional layer with a 3×3 kernel size, using Batch Normalization and ReLU

Non-linearity, followed by a MaxPooling operation. This module transforms the images from the format of $299 \times 299 \times 3$, at the input, to the format of $18 \times 18 \times 92$, at the output. The first two numbers are the dimension of the image, while the last is the number of channels. While starting with images of size 299×299 and 3 color channels, at the end the image is of size 18×18 and 92 abstract representation channels.

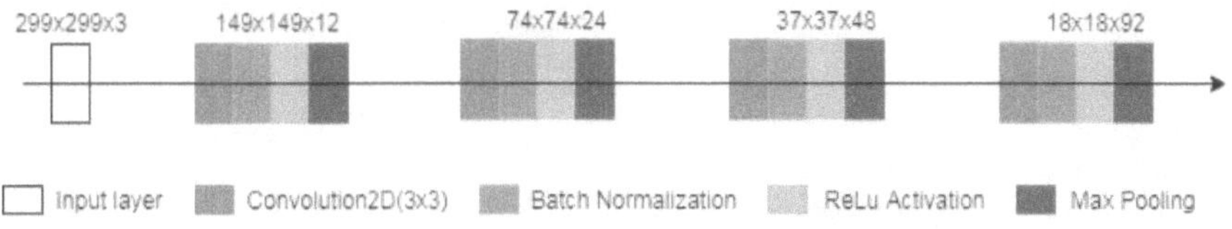

Figure 4.8: Diagram of the Feature extraction module.

In the end, the feature extraction module is connected to an alternative classification module, Figure 4.9. The alternative classification module is made of a Convolutional layer with a 3×3 kernel size, MaxPooling and ends on a GlobalAveragePooling with Softmax non-linearity for the classification.

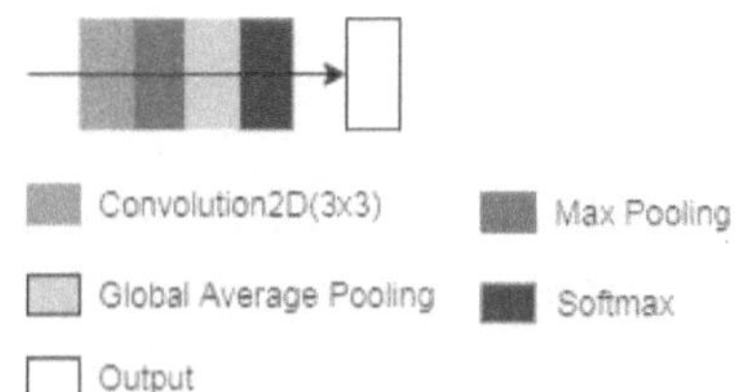

Figure 4.9: Diagram of the alternative Classification module.

In the Convolutional layer, the number of features are reduced to that of the same number as the target variables, 5 for the skin lesion classification learning task, while the GlobalAverage-Pooling layer reduces the dimension of the image. This results in the data taking the format of $1 \times 1 \times 5$, or a vector with 5 elements. This vector is fed to the Softmax non-linearity layer which outputs the probability of the instance belonging to each target variable. This probability is organized such that if the probabilities of all target variables of a learning task were to be added, a 100% is obtained. This module is used when a fusion is not performed.

To handle multiple inputs from different modalities, such as images or metadata, the previous architecture needs to be expanded with a fusion module. The diagram of the fusion module can be seen on Figure 4.10. This module is made of a Concatenation layer, followed by three blocks of Dense layer with ReLU Non-linearity. The Concatenation layer is where the various data types are fused together through concatenation. The data at this point takes the format of a vector of varying size at the concatenation layer, the size of the following blocks depends on the fusion type.

To perform class-fusion, the above network, in addition to metadata, is then connected to a

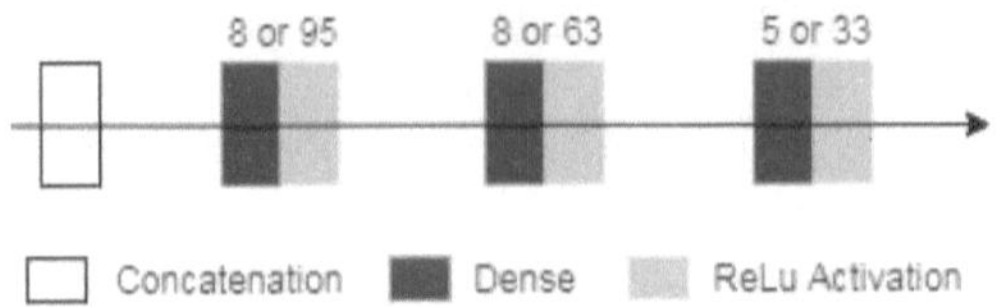

Figure 4.10: Diagram of the fusion module.

fusion module that then connects to a classification module, Figure 4.11. Lastly, the size of the blocks in this fusion module are 8, 8 and 5 respectively.

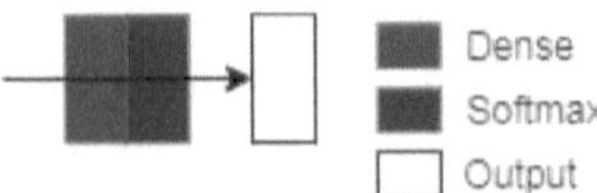

Figure 4.11: Diagram of the Classification module.

To perform feature-fusion, the features of each data type are processed to have the same dimension and fused. This requires that the classification module be removed from the first architecture. The image feature extraction module is connected to a GlobalAveragePooling layer that transforms the image data dimension from $18 \times 18 \times 92$ to $1 \times 1 \times 92$. This dimension is able to be concatenated with the metadata that has a dimension of 3. The image features and the metadata from the metadata input are then sent trough the fusion module, following into a classification module, Figure 4.11. In this case, the size of the blocks for the fusion module are 95, 63 and 33 respectively. 95 from the addition of the number of features from the images (92) and the number of metadata (3). The dimensions are reduced to 63 and 33 to be more suitable for the classification task.

Finally, to support the multitasking technique, the final classification modules needed to be changed/expanded into multitasking classification modules, Figure 4.12.

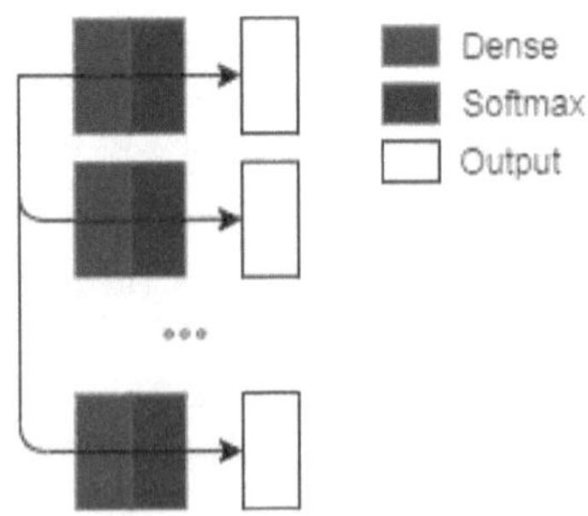

Figure 4.12: Diagram of the Multitask classification module.

The multitask classification module is simply several classification modules in parallel, one for each learning task. The above diagrams are simplified when demonstrating the built architectures for each of the experiments. Input data is represented as a white block, feature extraction module as a green block, fusion module as a yellow block, alternative classification module as a purple block and classification module as a blue block. The GlobalAveragePooling layer placed between the feature extraction module and the fusion module, when feature-fusion is utilized, is represented by a red block.

4.5 Evaluation metrics

A model is created with each configuration of the architecture for each experiment. During training, the effects of utilizing different modalities and slightly different architectures are measured through the average loss and average accuracy scores obtained at the end of each epoch. The loss function used is the Sparse Categorical Crossentropy [42], represented in equation 4.1, with this being the function that guides the training of the model. The validation data is used at the end of each epoch. The same metrics are obtained, serving as a comparison point to the training metrics, providing an idea for if the model is improving or overfitting.

$$- \sum_{i=1}^{number of samples} (true\_label_i \times log(predicted\_label_i)) \tag{4.1}$$

For the test data, more metrics were obtained. First a multilabel confusion matrix is constructed with the predictions from the model and the true values. Since the Softmax function outputs the probability of the sample belonging to each of the classes, the class that is predicted is the class with the highest probability.

Various metrics are obtained from the multilabel confusion matrix. The global accuracy is the only metric not specific to any class, while Sensitivity (SEN), Specificity (SPC), F1-score, Area under the receiver operating characteristic (AUROC) and Receiver Operating Characteristic (ROC) curve are obtained for each class. To calculate these metrics for each class, the one-vs-all method is used. This method takes turns placing each class as the positive class, with all of the other as the single negative class, allowing for the direct application of the formulas of each metric. AUROC is often used as a replacement for the accuracy metric as both give an idea of how accurate a model is. However, AUROC is a representation of the True positive rate (Sensitivity) with respect to the False Positive Rate. Despite this, accuracy is still obtained to have an overview of the overall performance of the model. The ROC curve allows the observation and choice of a trade off between Sensitivity and False Positive Rate.

With so many metrics used, deciding if an experiment is better than another requires significant examination. To simplify this, the average of SEN, SPC, F1-score and AUROC is calculated. The averaging of the metrics allows for a quick comparison. However, the average metrics only show the overall performance of the each experiment, with some obtaining the best results in individual classes or metrics.

4.6 Experiments

A total of eleven experiments were conducted to better understand the impact that the aforementioned techniques and the fusing of multiple modalities can have on skin lesion classification. Bias such as obtaining a higher sensitivity for malignant cancers is preferred in this domain, as the danger from not discovering cancerous lesions is considerably higher than incorrectly diagnosing a benign lesion. However, these biases were not introduced, as this work focuses on understanding the effects of the techniques and the various modalities. The experiments are summarised in Table 4.2. The table contains the experiments, the techniques used and with whom the experiment is comparable to.

Table 4.2: List of experiments, the techniques used and nearest comparable experiments.

#	Experiments	Class-fusion	Feature-fusion	Multitask	Comparable
exp1	Img				
exp2	ImgMd_CF	X			Img exp1
exp3	Img_MT7pts			X	Img exp1
exp4	ImgMd_CF_TransfL7pts	X			ImgMd_CF exp2 Img_MT7pts exp3
exp5	Img_MtMd			X	Img exp1 Img_MT7pts exp3
exp6	ImgMd_CF_TransfLMd	X			ImgMd_CF exp2 ImgMd_CF_TransfL7pts exp4 Img_MtMd exp5
exp7	ImgMd_FF		X		Img exp1 ImgMd_CF exp2
exp8	ImgMd_FF_MT7pts		X	X	ImgMd_CF exp2 ImgMd_FF exp7
exp9	2Img_FF_MT7pts		X	X	Img_MT7pts exp3 ImgMd_FF_MT7pts exp8
exp10	2ImgMd_FF_MT7pts		X	X	Img_MT7pts exp3 ImgMd_FF_MT7pts exp8 2Img_FF_MT7pts exp9
exp11	2ImgMd_CombFF_MT7pts		X	X	Img_MT7pts exp3 ImgMd_FF_MT7pts exp8 2ImgMd_FF_MT7pts exp10

The model of every experiment has the same hyperparameters and training epochs. The Learning Rate (LR), decay, momentum and epochs were investigated to find values that best supported the experiments. To ensure that the models are initialized with the same random weights, a seed is used at the time of their creation. The images used as input are all RGB color with size 299×299. Experiments 1 through 8 have a model trained separately for each image type: clinical and dermoscopic.

4.6.1 Img: Clinical/Dermoscopic Image (exp1)

In this experiment a simple model is designed. Its performance is used as the baseline from which the following experiments can be compared to. The architecture of this model can be observed in Figure 4.13. It is made of a feature extraction module connected to an alternative classification module. The input of the network is an image, the learning task is the skin lesion classification, with five classes: BCC, NEV, MEL, MISC and SK.

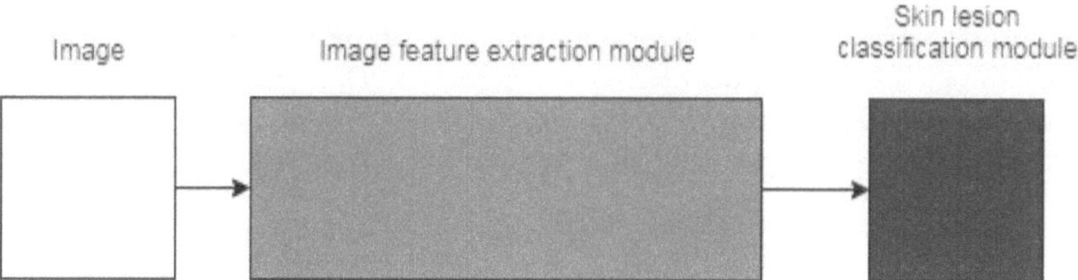

Figure 4.13: Diagram of the first experiment architecture.

4.6.2 ImgMd_CF: Clinical/Dermoscopic Image and Metadata Class-Fusion (exp2)

Can the results improve if the images are fused with metadata? In this experiment the multimodal aspect is introduced, with Image and metadata being fused through class-fusion?

The architecture of the model, shown in Figure 4.14, is made of a Feature extraction module connected to an alternative classification module. This module, in addition to a metadata input layer, is then connected to a class-fusion module, finishing in a classification module. The input of the network is an image **and metadata,** with the learning task being the skin lesion classification.

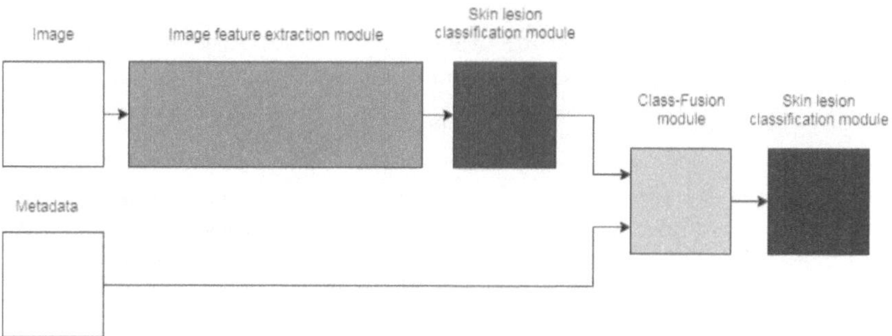

Figure 4.14: Diagram of the second experiment architecture.

4.6.3 Img_MT7pts: Clinical/Dermoscopic Image Multitask 7-points (exp3)

Can multitasking the categories of the 7-points checklist, in addition to the skin lesion classification, improve the results of the skin lesion classification?

This experiment differs slightly from the previous one, unlike the previous experiment where the fusion of multiple modalities was analysed, this experiment investigates the multitasking approach.

The architecture of the model, shown in Figure 4.15, is made of a Feature extraction module connected to a Multitask alternative classification module. The input of the network is an image. **Several learning tasks were performed simultaneously**, these being the skin lesion classification and the categories of the 7-point checklist, resulting in eight learning tasks.

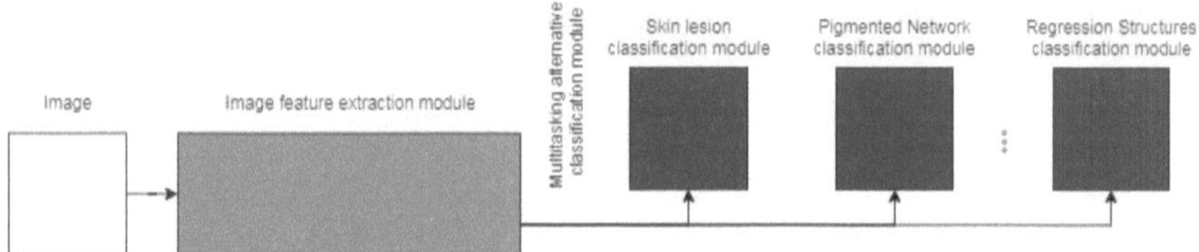

Figure 4.15: Diagram of the third experiment architecture.

4.6.4 ImgMd_CF_TransfL7pts: Clinical/Dermoscopic Image and Metadata Class-Fusion with Transfer Learning of multitask 7-points pre-training (exp4)

What is the impact of pre-training portions of the model with the multitasking of the 7-points?

This experiment utilizes the previous one, transferring the knowledge (weights and bias) of its feature extraction module and alternative classification module. This investigates what happens if the model is pre-trained on some modalities. The model is sequentially trained to the modalities, rather than being exposed to all of them at the start.

The architecture of the model, shown in Figure 4.16, is made of a Feature extraction module connected to an Alternative classification module. **This module is loaded with the knowledge from experiment** exp3. When loaded, this, together with a metadata input layer, is then connected to a class-fusion module, finishing in a Classification module. The input of the network is an image and metadata, with the learning task being the skin lesion classification.

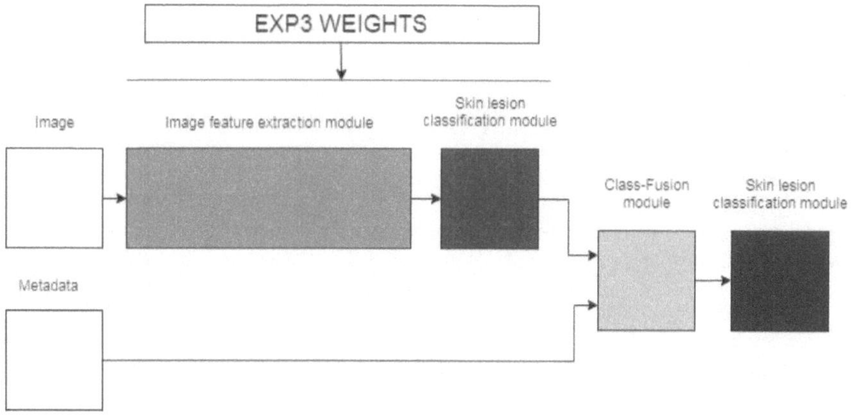

Figure 4.16: Diagram of the fourth experiment architecture.

4.6.5 Img_MtMd: Clinical/Dermoscopic Image Multitask Metadata (exp5)

What is the result of predicting the metadata through multitasking, rather than fusing it with the other modalities?

This experiment is similar to the Img_MT7pts experiment exp3, the difference stemming from multitasking with metadata rather than the categories of the 7-points checklist. This experiment investigates if predicting the metadata through multitasking would produce good results, rather than using it as an input.

The architecture of the model, shown in Figure 4.17, is made of a Feature extraction module connected to a Multitask alternative classification module. The input of the network is an image . Several Learning tasks were performed simultaneously, these being the skin lesion classification and **the metadata, resulting in four learning tasks**.

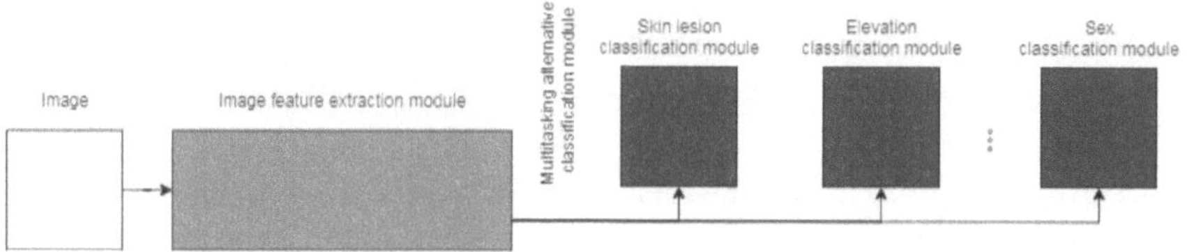

Figure 4.17: Diagram of the fifth experiment architecture.

4.6.6 ImgMd_CF_TransfLMd: Clinical/Dermoscopic Image and Metadata Class-Fusion with Transfer Learning of multitask Metadata pre-train (exp6)

Could pre-training parts of the model in metadata lead to a better fusion with metadata?

This experiment investigates if it is possible to bridge the gap between the various modalities by pre-training portions of the model with multitasking of those modalities. Equivalent to the ImgMd_CF_TransfL7pts experiment exp4, it replaces the 7-points for metadata.

The architecture of the model, shown in Figure 4.18, is made of a Feature extraction module connected to an Alternative classification module. This module is **loaded with the knowledge from experiment exp5**. When loaded, this, together with a metadata input layer, is then connected to a class-fusion module, finishing in a Classification module. The input of the network is an image and metadata, with the learning task being the skin lesion classification.

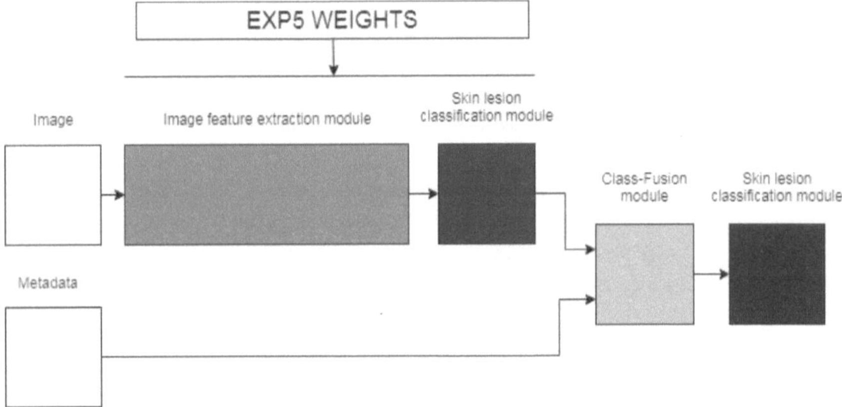

Figure 4.18: Diagram of the sixth experiment architecture.

This was the last experiment involving the transferring of knowledge (transfer learning) and sequential training of the model with various modalities (pre-training).

4.6.7 ImgMd_FF: Clinical/Dermoscopic Image and Metadata Feature-Fusion (exp7)

Would the results improve if the fusion of the modalities were to be performed at the features (feature-fusion)?

This experiment investigates the differences between class-fusion and feature-fusion. It serves as a bridge between experiments performed with class-fusion and experiments performed with feature-fusion. Feature-fusion is also used in Kawahara et al [44] work.

The architecture of the model, shown in Figure 4.19, is made of a Feature extraction module connected to a GlobalAveragePooling layer. This module, in addition to a metadata input layer, is then connected to a **feature-fusion module**, finishing in a Classification module. The input of the network is an image and metadata, with the learning task being the skin lesion classification.

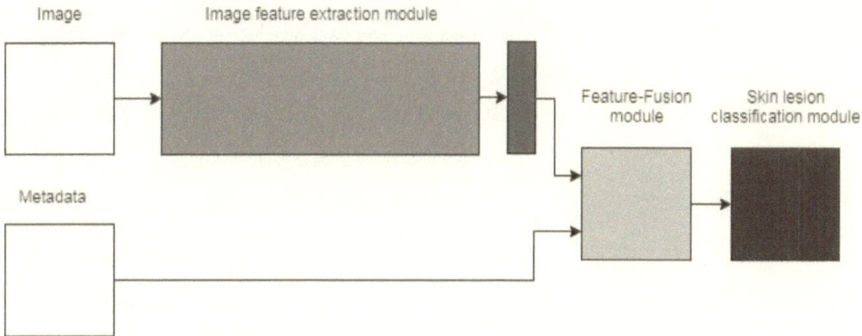

Figure 4.19: Diagram of the seventh experiment architecture.

4.6.8 ImgMd_FF_MT7pts: Clinical/Dermoscopic Image and Metadata Feature-Fusion Multitasking 7-points (exp8)

Will multitasking the the categories of the 7-points improve the results obtained by feature-fusion images and metadata?

This experiment, along with experiments 3 and 10, is the execution of one of the 5 simultaneous combinations performed in [44]. In this case, an image and metadata are feature-fused and the categories of the 7-points are multitasked. The effects of multitasking on top of feature fusion are investigated, as well as serving as a comparison to experiment exp11.

The architecture of the model, shown in Figure 4.20, is made of a Feature extraction module connected to a GlobalAveragePooling layer. This module, in addition to a metadata input layer, is then connected to a **feature-fusion module, finishing in a Multiclass classification module.** The input of the network is an image and metadata, with several Learning tasks being performed simultaneously, these being the skin lesion classification and the categories of the 7-point checklist, resulting in in eight learning tasks.

4.6.9 2Img_FF_MT7pts: Both Images Feature-Fusion Multitasking 7-points (exp9)

What would be the results of the feature-fusion of both images, with multitasking the categories of the 7-points?

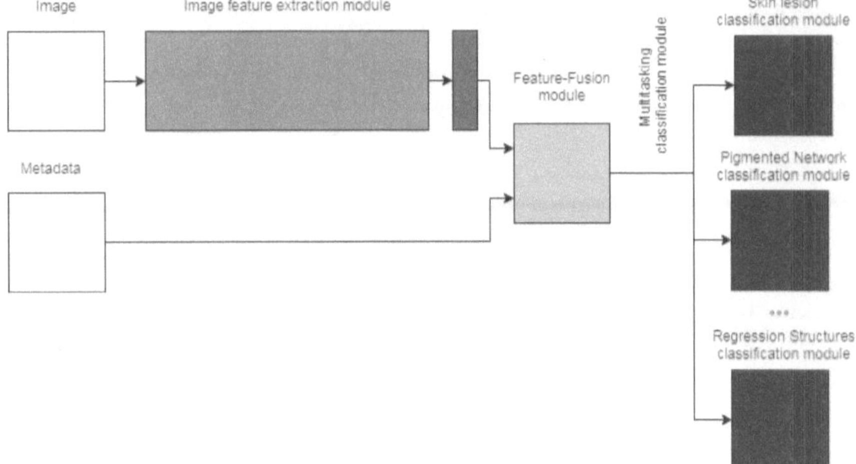

Figure 4.20: Diagram of the eighth experiment architecture.

This experiment investigates the effect of feature-fusing both types of image. This experiment is situated before using all of the data to provide an idea of what the results would look like if just clinical and dermoscopic images were fused.

The architecture of the model, shown in Figure 4.21, is made of two Feature extraction modules, each connected to a GlobalAveragePooling layer. **A module for clinical images and the other for dermoscopic images**. Both modules are then connected to a feature-fusion module, finishing in a Multiclass classification module. The input of the network consists of two images (clinical and dermoscopic), with several Learning tasks being performed simultaneously, these being the skin lesion classification and the categories of the 7-point checklist, resulting in in eight learning tasks.

4.6.10 2ImgMd_FF_MT7pts: Both Images Metadata Feature-Fusion Multitasking 7-points (exp10)

What is the result of feature-fusion all of the available modalities, with multitasking the categories of the 7-points?

This experiment shows the effect of using: all modalities, clinical images, dermoscopic images and metadata. The modalities are fused through feature-fusion. This experiment is the full combinations of the model in [44].

The architecture of the model, shown in Figure 4.22, is made of two Feature extraction modules, each connected to a GlobalAveragePooling layer. A module for clinical images and the other for dermoscopic images. **Both modules and a metadata input layer are** then

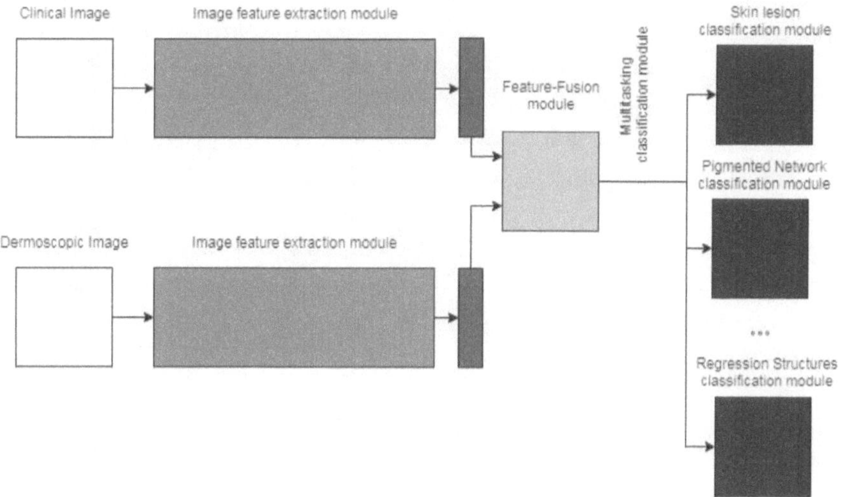

Figure 4.21: Diagram of the ninth experiment architecture.

connected to a feature-fusion module, finishing in a Multiclass classification module. The input of the network are two RGB color images and metadata, with several Learning tasks being performed simultaneously, these being the skin lesion classification and the categories of the 7-point checklist, resulting in eight learning tasks.

4.6.11 2ImgMd_CombFF_MT7pts: Both Images Metadata Combinations of Feature-Fusion Multitasking 7-points (exp11)

Could multitasking a multitude of combinations in the same model obtain better results?

In this experiment, an adaptation of the architecture from Kawahara in [44] is utilized. The architecture includes several combinations of fusions, each leading to multitask classifications. The combinations include the dermoscopic image combination, a dermoscopic image and metadata combination, a dermoscopic image, clinical image and metadata combination, a clinical image and metadata combination, and a clinical image combination. The main difference between this model and Kawahara's model is the CNN used to extract features from the images. Kawahara used a pre-trained deeper network architecture than was used in this work.

The architecture of the model, shown in Figure 4.23, is made of two Feature extraction modules, each connected to a GlobalAveragePooling layer. A module for clinical images and the other for dermoscopic images. Both modules and a metadata input layer are then connected to several feature-fusion modules. One feature fusion for clinical images only (similar to Clinical exp3), another for clinical and metadata (similar to Clinical exp8), other for clinical, dermoscopic and metadata (all data, similar to exp10), dermoscopic and metadata (similar to Dermoscopic exp8),

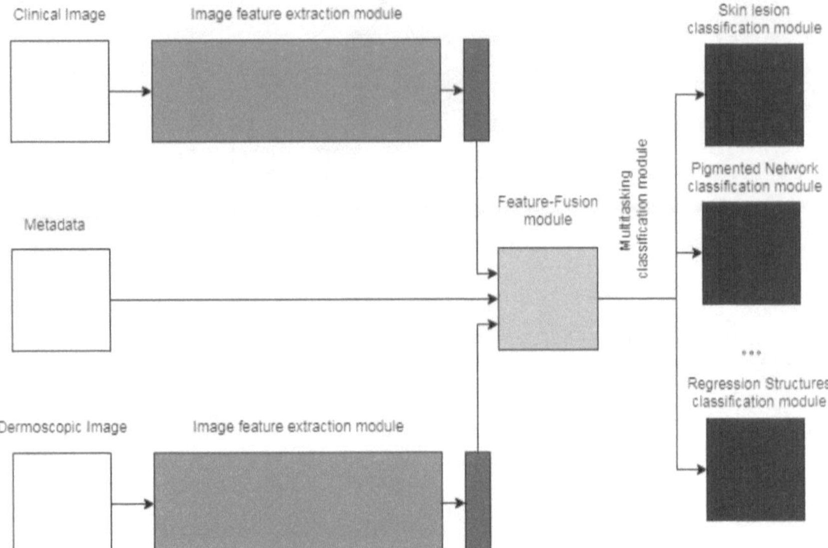

Figure 4.22: Diagram of the tenth experiment architecture.

and in dermoscopic only fusion (similar to Dermoscopic exp3), resulting in in five fusions. Each of these fusions is connected to a Multiclass classification module. The input of the network are two RGB color images and metadata, with several Learning tasks being performed in each fusion simultaneously, these being the skin lesion classification and the categories of the 7-point checklist, resulting in eight learning tasks for each combination of modalities, resulting in forty learning tasks total.

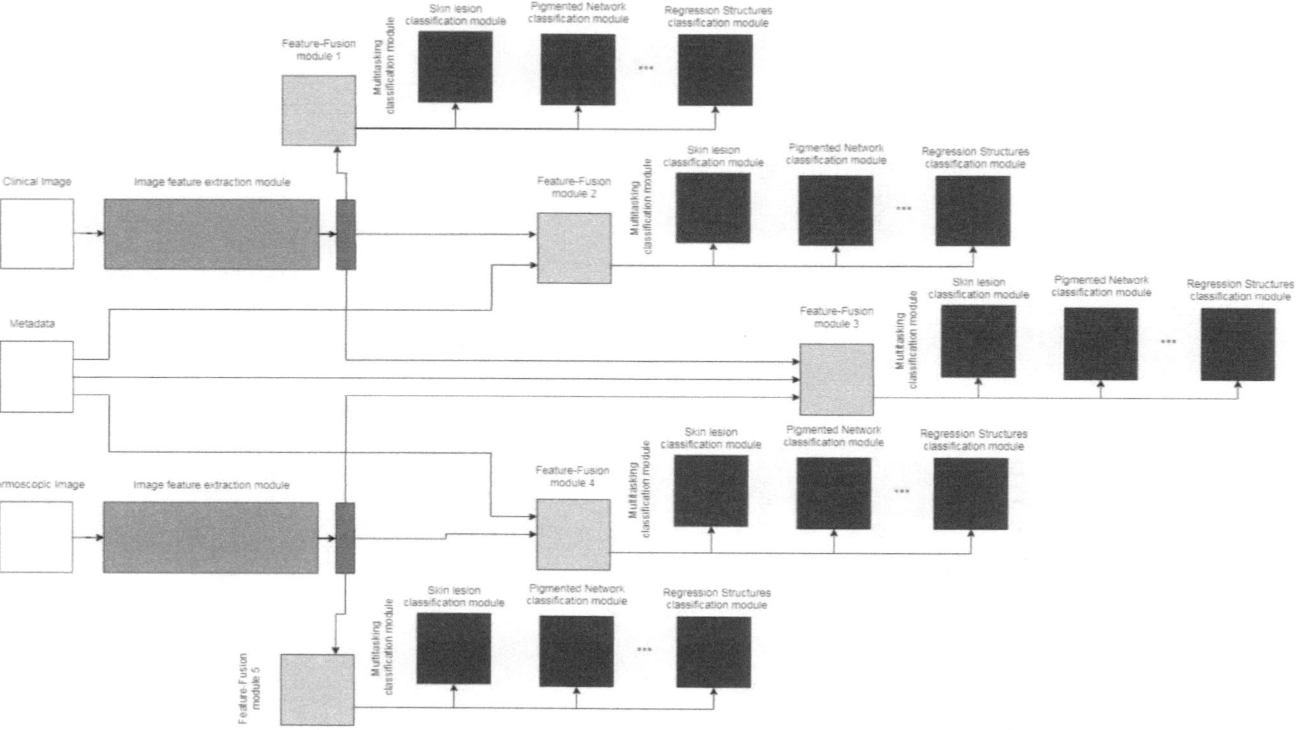

Figure 4.23: Diagram of the eleventh experiment architecture.

Chapter 5

Results and analysis

This chapter presents the results obtained for the different models that were described in the previous chapter. Focus is placed on the relevant information found in the results, the full range of the results obtained can be seen on the Appendix A.

The chapter starts by discussing about preliminary results to adjust hyperparameters, Section 5.1. Then the results followed by a small discussion of each of the eleven experiments are shown in Sections res1 through res11. The chapter ends with a summary of the results.

5.1 Hyperparameters

Several tuning experiments were performed to set the learning rate. Regarding other hyperparameters, no further tests were performed.

The impact of the Learning Rate (LR) over the network was analysed. In cases where a high LR ($1e^{-3}$) was utilized, the model generates large variations of the loss and accuracy, see Figure 5.1.

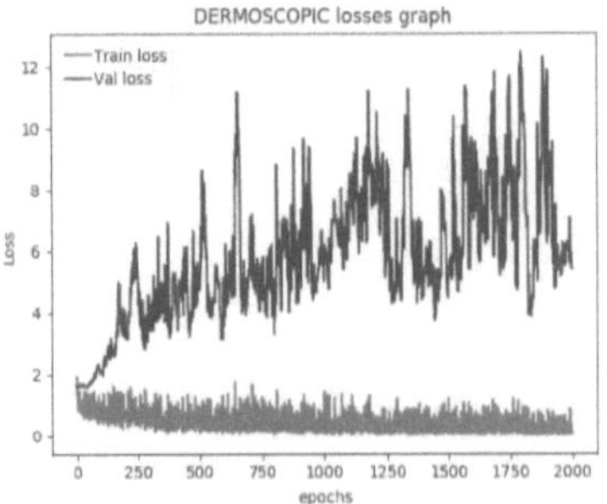
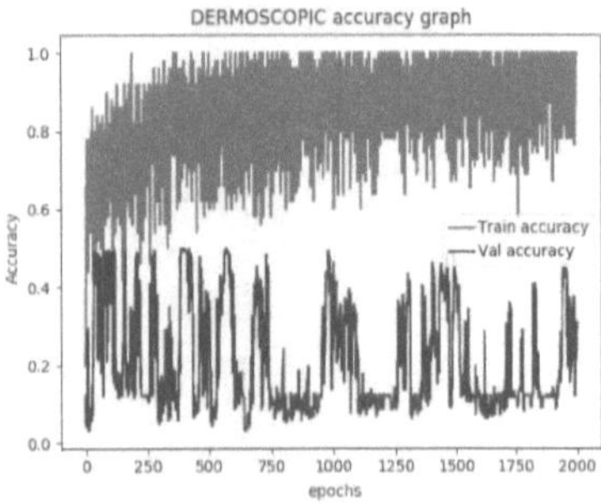

Figure 5.1: High LR, loss and accuracy obtained over the course of training for 2000 epochs.

Low LR ($1e^{-9}$), on the other hand, resulted in far smaller differences in the loss and accuracy between epochs, see Figure 5.2.

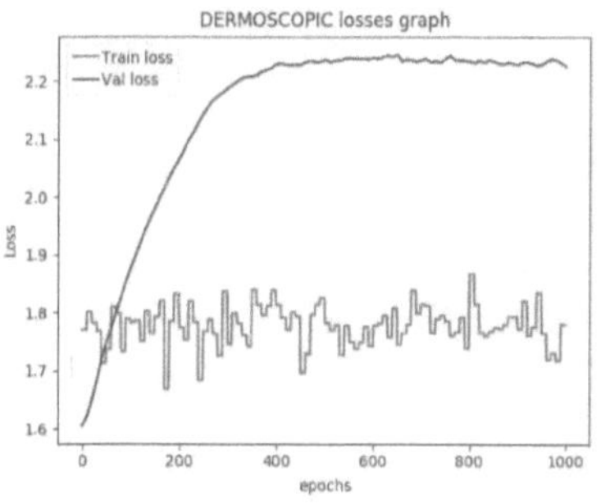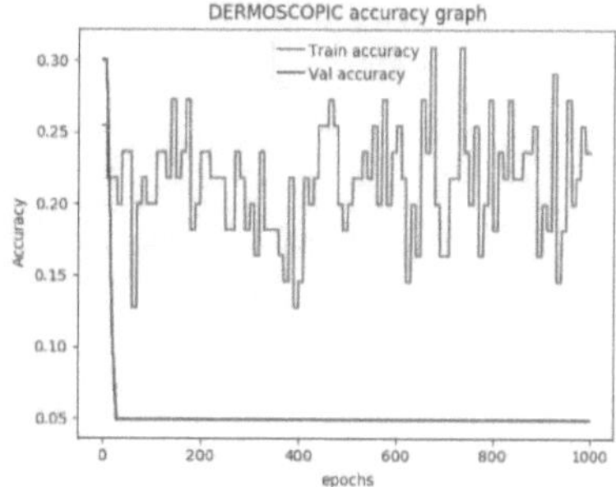

Figure 5.2: Low LR, loss and accuracy obtained over the course of training for 1000 epochs.

As such, high LR enables the model to learn faster, but does not allow to reach a minimum loss. While low LR forces the model to make small changes, learning at a slower pace but with more focus on whichever minimum it currently is situated. A balanced approach of LR is best suited to the training of a model. Starting with a high value so that the model can learn faster and ending with a low value to fine-tune the model, however attention was paid so that the model did not overfit with the low LR.

Different decays caused differences in the training, as can be seen in Figure 5.3 through Figure 5.6. 4 decays are investigated, low decay, high decay, calculated decay and linear LR. The starting LR value is always $1e^{-3}$ for all experiments.

Figure 5.3 shows training with a high decay ($1e^{-1}$). The LR lowers so quickly that it decreases an order of magnitude in the first epoch. Only a small number of epochs benefit from a high LR, resulting in the model not having enough time to find a best minimum Loss.

Figure 5.4 shows training with low decay ($1e^{-10}$), the decrease in the LR is so low that it basically does not change during the training. Due to this the model trains quicker, but does not converge, with large variations in the validation loss.

Figure 5.5 shows training with a decay calculated such that it would end on a predetermined LR over the course of the training. This makes it so that the training does not utilize too low of a LR, while allowing the decay to naturally transition from the starting LR to the ending LR.

Lastly, Figure 5.6 shows training with a linear LR, shifting from the starting LR to the ending LR. This training enables the model to spend more time with a higher LR, enabling it to find a better minimum before converging, leading to the best validation loss and accuracy values.

The hyperparameters are the same for every model in the experiments, meaning that each model as the same momentum, kept at the default value of 0.9. training is done over 500 epochs,

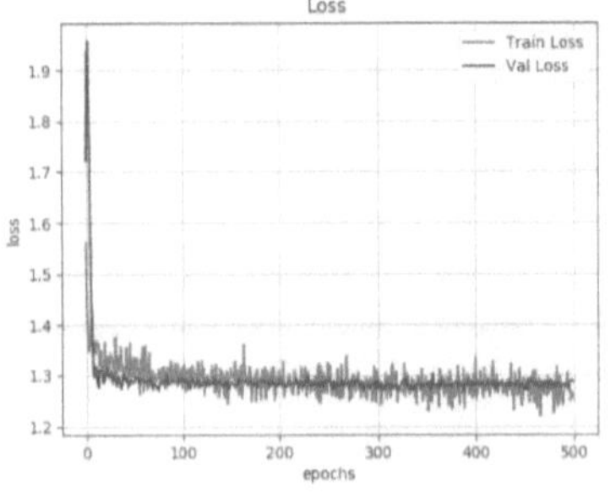

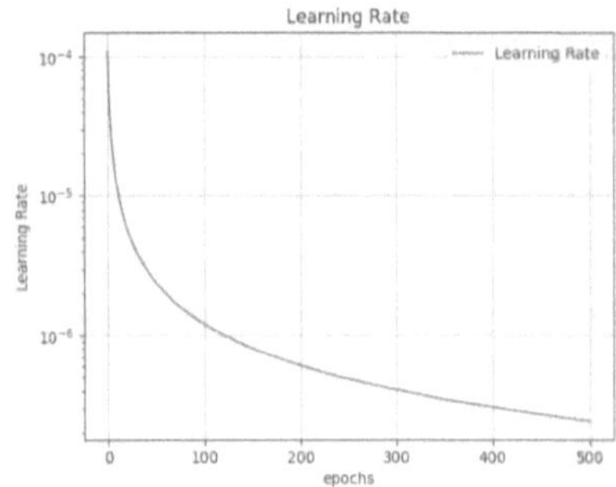

(a) Train and validation loss for the high decay model.

(b) LR for the high decay model.

Figure 5.3: Train and validations loss acquired during training and the progression of the LR in a model with a high decay.

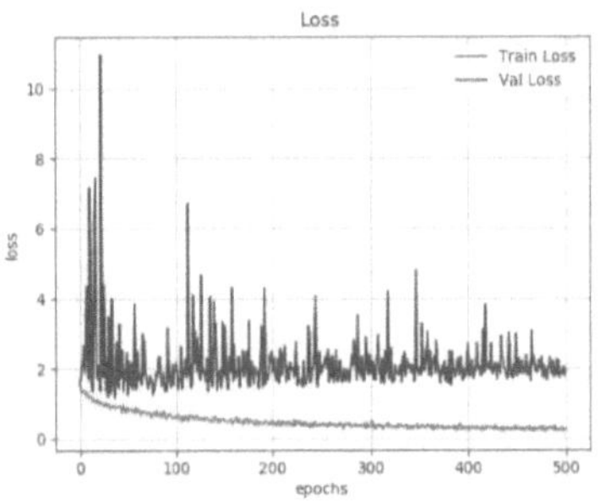

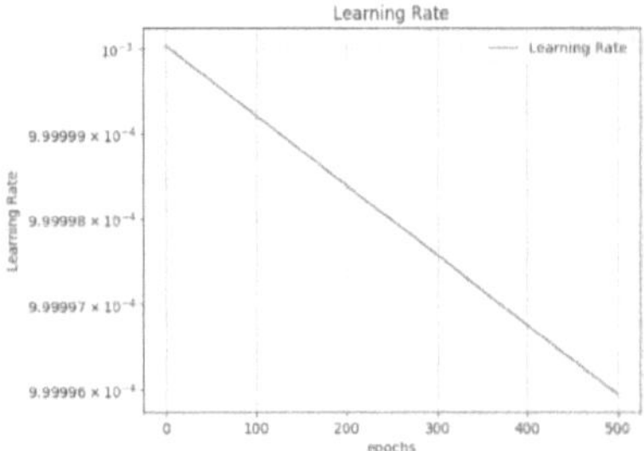

(a) Train and validation loss for the low decay model.

(b) LR for the low decay model.

Figure 5.4: Train and validations loss acquired during training and the progression of the LR in a model with a low decay.

as this value proved to be a good balance between the converging of the loss and overfitting. Lastly, the decay is the linear LR, with the LR starting at 1e-3 and ending at 1e-4, as these values lead to better results.

5.2 Img (exp1)

Utilizing the models detailed in Subsection exp1, this first experiment establishes a baseline that the following experiments can compare to. A clinical baseline and a dermoscopic baseline are established with a model trained on clinical images and a model trained on dermoscopic images,

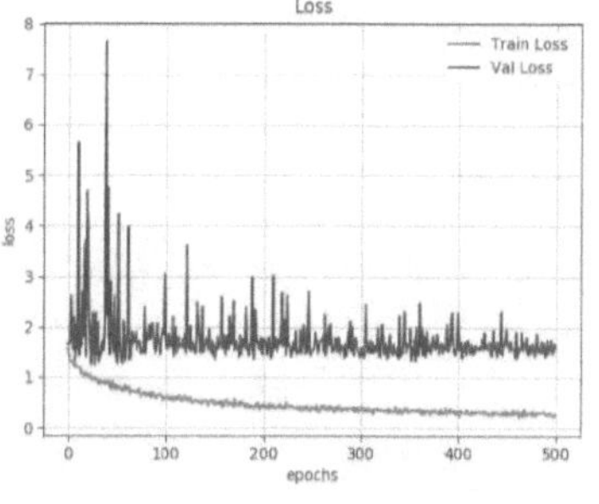
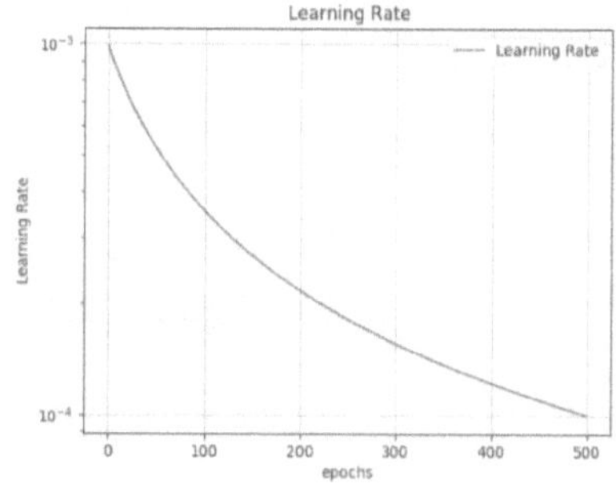

(a) Train and validation loss for the calculated decay model.

(b) LR for the calculated decay model.

Figure 5.5: Train and validations loss acquired during training and the progression of the LR in a model with a calculated decay.

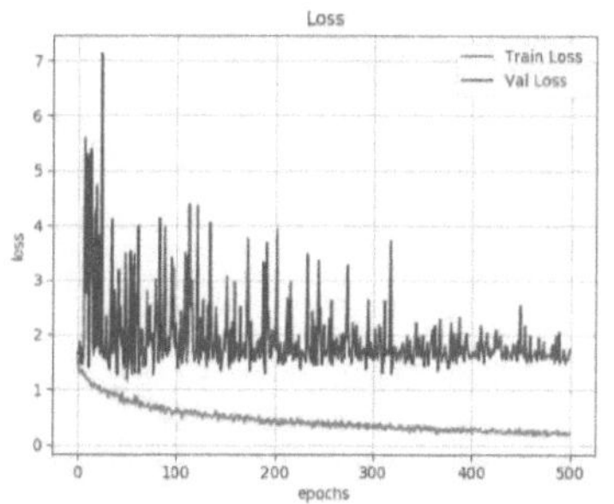
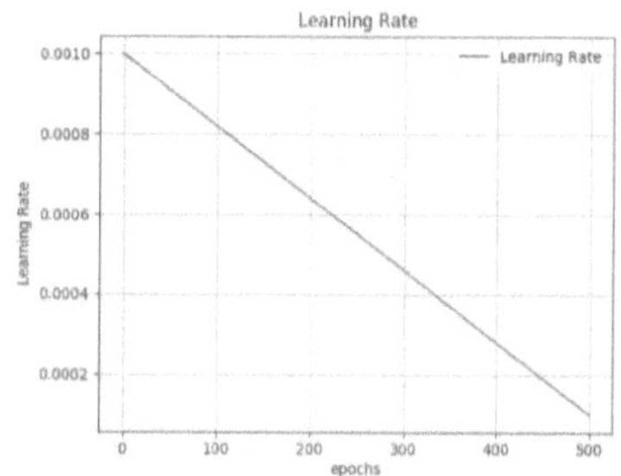

(a) Train and validation loss for the linear LR model.

(b) LR for the linear LR model.

Figure 5.6: Train and validations loss acquired during training and the progression of the LR in a model with a linear LR.

respectively.

During the training (Figure 5.7), both models converge their training loss and improve the training accuracy. The validation loss increases to a certain point, before decreasing and plateauing, while the validation accuracy slightly improves. The model trained on clinical images (CImg) shows the validation loss forming a curve (Figure 5.7a), increasing from 1.8 to an averaged maximum of ≈ 2.8, at the 340 epoch, before starting to decrease to ≈ 2.5. The validation accuracy is constantly increasing from 0.2 to 0.41. The model trained on dermoscopic images (DImg) obtains better values in both loss and accuracy than the CImg (Figure 5.7b) while showing a similar progression, reaching ≈ 1.9 validation loss and ≈ 0.6 validation accuracy.

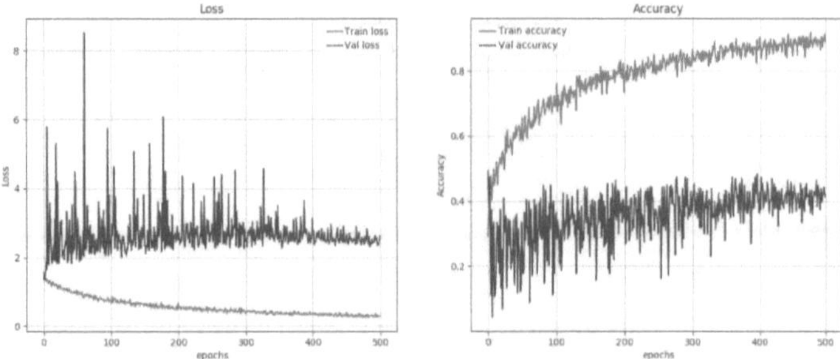

(a) Loss and accuracy metric scores for the model trained on clinical images.

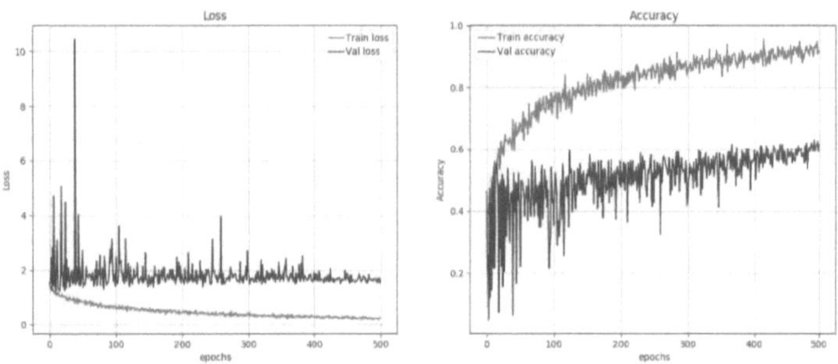

(b) Loss and accuracy metric scores for the model trained on dermoscopic images.

Figure 5.7: Loss and validation metric scores for the baseline models. Figures on the left show the training (red) and validation (blue) loss. The figures on the right show the training (red) and validation (blue) accuracy.

The Receiver Operating Characteristic (ROC) curves shown in Figure 5.8 were obtained from the test set, these show the performance of the models in each class. The ROC curves show that, in general, better results are obtained from the dermoscopic images. The performance of the model for each class depends on the type of image, with CImg obtaining the best performances from the clinical images for, in descending order according to the AUROC, the Miscellaneous (MISC), Nevus (NEV), Basal Cell Carcinoma (BCC), Melanoma (MEL) and Seborrheic Keratosis (SK) classes while the DImg acquires the best performances from the dermoscopic images for the MISC, BCC/SK, NEV and MEL classes.

The multilabel confusion matrix shown in figure 5.9 was obtained with the test set, showing the matching between the predicted labels from each model, using the best probability, and the true labels of the samples. The color of the multilabel confusion matrix indicates the percentage of true samples present in that cell. The color varies in the ascending order from red to blue.

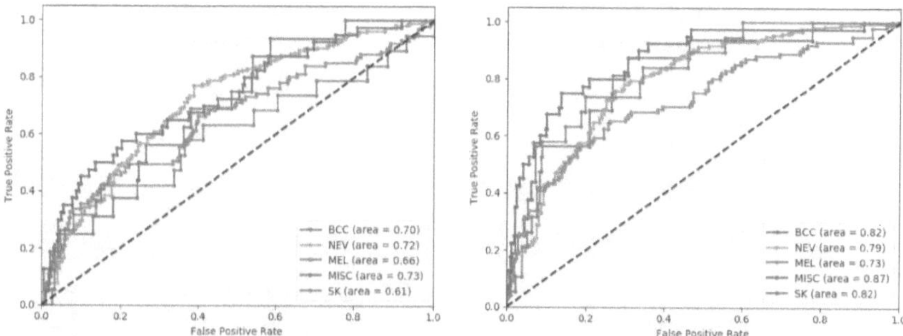

(a) ROC curves for the model trained on clinical images.

(b) ROC curves for the model trained on dermoscopic images.

Figure 5.8: ROC curves for the baseline models.

The multilabel confusion matrix on the clinical images (Figure 5.9a) does not show a good classification for the BCC, MISC and SK classes, the model correctly classifying less than half of the true samples for each class, with the remaining samples being predicted as another class. Furthermore, the BCC and SK classes have a considerable number of false predictions, mostly NEV and MEL samples. The model achieves the highest performances with NEV and MEL, as can be observed by the color of their diagonal cell, both having mostly half of their true samples correctly classified. It is noticeable that NEV and MEL are difficult to differentiate, as close to half, 70 samples, of NEV were misclassified as MEL.

The multilabel confusion matrix on dermoscopic images (Figure 5.9b) presents better results than the matrix for the CImg. MEL has a similar number of correctly classified samples, but with a lower number of predictions. NEV sees an increase in the number of predictions, with the extra predictions being almost all correctly classified samples (true positives), as indicated by the higher number in the diagonal cell. As there are fewer NEV samples being mislabeled as MEL, this suggests that the model differentiates better between NEV and MEL. The number of correctly classified samples for the MISC class increases, but so does the number of predictions, leading to a higher Sensitivity (SEN) with a lower Specificity (SPC) value, as seen in Table 5.1.

Table 5.1 shows the obtained values for various metric scores. Global accuracy is shown for all classes. SEN, SPC, F1-score and Area under the receiver operating characteristic (AUROC) is shown for each class. And the average of each metric is shown in the last row. Test metric scores tables like this one are presented for every experiment henceforth, with the left side belonging to models trained on clinical images and the right side belonging to models trained on dermoscopic images when such cases occur.

From it, several conclusions can be drawn on top of the multilabel confusion matrix. The global accuracy is high, compared with some SEN and F1-scores, due to the NEV and MEL classes. These classes have the highest number of samples and the model performed better on

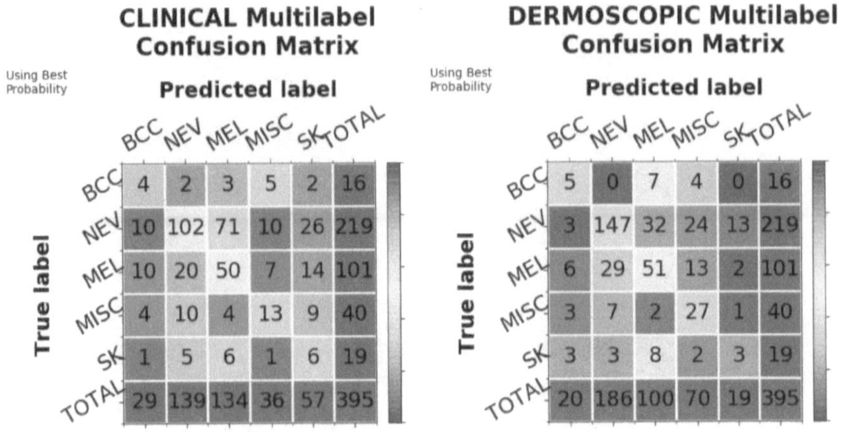

(a) Multilabel confusion matrix for the model trained on clinical images. (b) Multilabel confusion matrix for the model trained on dermoscopic images.

Figure 5.9: Multilabel confusion matrix for the baseline models.

them, resulting an overall higher global accuracy. A common situation is the high value of SPC for every class. This is due to the one-vs-all approach used to calculate each metric. This ends with four of the five classes being grouped under a "false" class, elevating the SPC value to near the best of 1, especially in the classes with a lower number of samples such as BCC or SK.

For the CImg, the global accuracy is 0.44. The SEN for NEV and MEL is the highest, at 0.47 and 0.5 respectively, while the BCC class has the lowest value at 0.25. The F1-score generally obtained values lower than the SEN, with NEV and MISC being the only classes with higher F1 scores. The lowest values were that of 0.18 and 0.16 from the BCC and SK classes respectively, while the NEV class obtained the highest value of 0.57. The AUROC metric is slightly different from the other metrics as its scores fluctuate around the 0.7 score, with the SK class having the lowest AUROC at 0.61.

The DImg shows a higher global accuracy, with a general increase in all of the metric scores. There are however some values that remain similar, such as the SEN of MEL and F1 of SK, and others that are lower, such as the SPC of MISC and SEN of SK. The changes in the MISC and SK classes are caused in part due to the change of the number of predicted samples. MISC sees an increase in the number of predictions, from 36 to 70, which leads to an increase in SEN and decrease in SPC. In the SK class, the opposite happens, as there are fewer predictions, lower SEN and higher SPC. The largest difference between these two classes is their F1-score, as the MISC class improves to 0.49, while the SK class keeps at the same 0.16. This F1-score supports the theory that the performance of the model over the MISC class improved, despite the decrease in SPC, but the performance over the SK class remains unchanged, only that the model had fewer samples to work with after predicting the other, better performing, classes.

EXP		CImg					DImg				
		ACC	SEN	SPC	F1	AUROC	ACC	SEN	SPC	F1	AUROC
1	BCC	0.44	0.25	0.93	0.18	0.7	0.59	0.31	0.96	0.28	0.82
	NEV		0.47	0.79	0.57	0.72		0.67	0.78	0.73	0.79
	MEL		**0.50**	0.71	0.43	0.66		**0.50**	0.83	0.51	0.73
	MISC		0.33	**0.94**	0.34	0.73		0.68	**0.88**	0.49	0.87
	SK		**0.32**	0.86	**0.16**	0.61		**0.16**	0.96	**0.16**	0.82
	AVG		0.374	0.846	0.336	0.684		0.464	0.882	0.434	0.806

To summarize, the baselines shows that dermoscopic images are better at differentiating between the lesions. This result was expected since dermoscopic images intrinsically carry more information about the lesion. What is noticeable is that the SK class seems to be less affected by image type, as the changes to its metric scores can be justified by the number of samples predicted to it with the model having the same performance in the class.

5.3   ImgMd_CF (exp2)

The dataset contains metadata. This extra modality might contain useful information that helps the model to better differentiate between the classes. However, its introduction, following the model detailed in Subsection exp2, produced inconclusive results.

Table 5.2 shows that the model trained on clinical images (CImgMd_CF) obtained higher results compared with the CImg. Its global accuracy, along with the average SPC, F1 and AUROC increased, with only the average SEN decreasing by 0.002. The reason for these changes are observed in the results for the BCC class. The metric scores for BCC are all higher, however, the average SEN reduced due to the lower performance over the MEL and MISC classes. Both MEL and MISC have lower F1 and AUROC scores. Although the SPC of MISC is higher, the SEN increased a at lower rate. This effect is supported by the F1 metric, which results in an overall lower performance of the model on these classes. The model improves slightly in the performance over the NEV class. Obtaining a slight increase of SEN and F1-score, with a slight decrease in SPC and AUROC. The increase in F1 is larger than the loss in AUROC, resulting in an overall small improvement. The performance over the SK class, remains similar, as is indicated by the similar F1-score and AUROC values. There are changes in the SEN and SPC, but these changes can be justified with the change in the number of predictions, from 57 to 22, and obtaining similar performance.

On the other hand, the model trained on dermoscopic images (DImgMd_CF) performed worse than the DImg. The global accuracy, along with the average SPC, F1 and AUROC decreased. Again, the increase in the performance over the BCC class is seen. The performance over the SK class also increases, contrary to the CImgMd_CF where it is similar. On the other hand, the performances over NEV, MEL and MISC decreased, obtaining lower SEN, F1 and AUROC. Since the NEV and MEL classes contain a large portion of the samples, their lower performance leads to a lower global accuracy. As seen in the confusion matrix (Figure 5.10b), the model predicted too many samples as the MISC class. This resulted in more true positives, leading to a higher SEN, but the loss in SPC did not produce an overall gain in performance, as is supported by the lower F1-score and AUROC. The performance of the SK class ended up benefiting from the fusion of metadata and dermoscopic images, contrary to the CImgMd_CF, as all of its metric scores, except for the AUROC, increased.

Table 5.2: Test metric scores for the ImgMd_CF (exp2) experiment and its closest comparison, Img (exp1).

EXP		CImgMd_CF					DImgMd_CF				
		ACC	SEN	SPC	F1	AUROC	ACC	SEN	SPC	F1	AUROC
2	**BCC**	0.46	0.38	0.96	0.31	0.86	0.45	0.38	0.96	0.32	0.87
	NEV		**0.51**	0.76	**0.6**	0.71		0.42	0.80	0.53	0.68
	MEL		0.46	0.71	0.39	0.6		0.42	0.86	0.45	0.66
	MISC		0.35	0.86	0.27	0.67		**0.85**	0.67	0.36	0.83
	SK		0.16	0.95	**0.15**	**0.61**		**0.26**	0.98	**0.32**	0.82
	AVG		0.372	**0.848**	**0.344**	**0.69**		**0.466**	0.854	0.396	0.772
EXP		CImg					DImg				
1	BCC	0.44	0.25	0.93	0.18	0.7	0.59	0.31	0.96	0.28	0.82
	NEV		0.47	**0.79**	0.57	**0.72**		0.67	0.78	**0.73**	**0.79**
	MEL		**0.50**	0.71	0.43	0.66		0.50	0.83	**0.51**	**0.73**
	MISC		**0.33**	0.94	0.34	0.73		0.68	0.88	**0.49**	**0.87**
	SK		0.32	0.86	**0.16**	**0.61**		0.16	0.96	0.16	0.82
	AVG		**0.374**	0.846	0.336	0.684		0.464	**0.882**	**0.434**	**0.806**

From the multilabel confusion matrices shown in Figure 5.10, both models have a lower number of predictions in the SK class, with the number of predictions in the MISC class increasing. The DImgMd_CF especially overemphasized the MISC class, as it predicted a lot more samples than exists as MISC, 150 predictions to the 40 total true MISC samples. Lastly there is an increase in the number of predictions for the NEV class from the CImgMd_CF. An important occurrence is the lower performance over the MEL class by the CImgMd_CF (Figure 5.10a), as there are 4 less true positives, with 2 less predictions, a situation where there loss in true positives is higher than the loss in predictions.

The inclusion of metadata brings an improvement to the performance of the models on the BCC class, however there is a large negative impact in the performance in the other classes to achieve this.

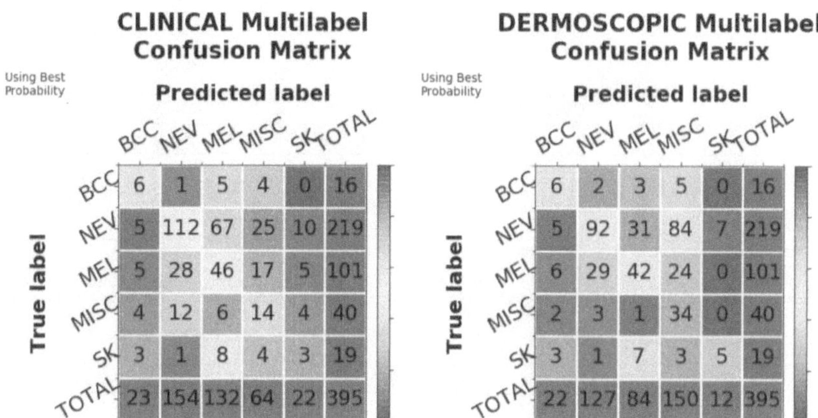

(a) Multilabel confusion matrix for the model trained on clinical images.

(b) Multilabel confusion matrix for the model trained on dermoscopic images.

Figure 5.10: Multilabel confusion matrices for the models of the second experiment.

5.4   Img_MT7pts (exp3)

By utilizing the models detailed in Subsection exp3, a simultaneous classification of the lesions and the categories of the 7-point checklist, i.e. multitasking, is performed, providing a small increase in global accuracy.

The metric scores, seen in Table 5.3, show that the model trained on clinical images (CImg_MT7pts) only slightly improved the global accuracy (+0.01), with the average metric scores all being lower than the CImg. The MEL class was the only class to improve, with all of the remaining classes having lower SEN and F1-score. The reason for the slightly higher global accuracy is due to the increase in the performance over MEL with a slight decrease in the performance over NEV. Regarding the SPC metric, the scores varied, there is an increase for the SK class, similar scores for the MISC class, and lower values for the BCC, NEV and MEL classes.

The model trained on dermoscopic images (DImg_MT7pts) performed better than the CImg_MT7pts. It obtained a small increase in average SEN and F1, in addition to the small increase of the global accuracy over the DImg. The performance of DImg_MT7pts over NEV, MEL and MISC was similar to DImg. The classes obtained different SPC and SEN scores but maintained similar F1-scores and AUROC. What improved was the performance over the SK class, increasing the SEN and F1, with similar SPC and AUROC. The performance over BCC lowered due to lower F1, AUROC and SEN, despite a higher SPC score.

Figure 5.11 shows the multilabel confusion matrix for the models of the third experiment.

Table 5.3: Test metric scores for the Img_MT7pts (exp3) experiment and its closest comparison, Img (exp1).

EXP		CImg_MT7pts					DImg_MT7pts				
		ACC	SEN	SPC	F1	AUROC	ACC	SEN	SPC	F1	AUROC
3	BCC		0.13	0.96	0.12	0.64		0.19	0.98	0.22	0.74
	NEV		0.46	0.77	0.56	0.69		0.71	0.70	0.73	0.79
	MEL	0.45	**0.65**	0.60	**0.46**	**0.68**	0.6	0.42	0.93	0.51	0.76
	MISC		0.23	0.94	0.26	0.7		0.8	0.83	0.48	0.87
	SK		0.11	0.95	0.10	0.56		**0.26**	0.95	**0.24**	0.82
	AVG		0.316	0.844	0.3	0.654		**0.476**	0.878	**0.436**	0.796
EXP		CImg					DImg				
1	BCC		0.25	0.93	0.18	0.7		**0.31**	0.96	**0.28**	0.82
	NEV		0.47	0.79	0.57	0.72		0.67	0.78	0.73	0.79
	MEL	0.44	0.50	**0.71**	0.43	0.66	0.59	0.50	0.83	0.51	0.73
	MISC		0.33	0.94	0.34	0.73		0.68	0.88	0.49	0.87
	SK		0.32	0.86	0.16	0.61		0.16	0.96	0.16	0.82
	AVG		**0.374**	**0.846**	**0.336**	**0.68**		0.464	**0.882**	0.434	**0.806**

The CImg_MT7pts predicts more samples in the MEL class, as can be observed in the multilabel confusion matrix, Figure 5.11a. MEL is the only class improving as of the large number of predictions in the class, there was an increase in 16 true positives in comparison with CImg (Figure 5.9a). However, of the additional 51 predictions, 35 were incorrectly classified as MEL. It is worth mentioning that, the number of true positives in NEV is similar to the baseline, 100 to 102 (CImg), despite a larger number of predictions in the NEV class, 141 to 139(CImg) . Another large misclassification occurs with the SK samples, as a large portion of these are misclassified as MEL.

The multilabel confusion matrix for the DImg_MT7pts (Figure 5.11b) has a higher number of predicted samples for NEV and MISC, compared to the DImg (Figure 5.9b), resulting in higher true positives. Contrary to the CImg_MT7pts, MEL sees a decrease in the number of predicted samples, with lower true positives, 51 (DImg) to 42. For this model, it is the BCC class that had a large number of its samples misclassified as MISC.

Multitasking the categories from the 7-point checklist seems to favour the large classes of NEV and MEL. This results in higher accuracy due to the small increase in performance in the larger classes. However, both models perform worse for the BCC class than the baseline.

5.5 ImgMd_CF_TransfL7pts (exp4)

Transferring the knowledge (weights and bias) from the third experiment, the model described in Subsection exp4 is used to investigate the results from pre-training portions of a model.

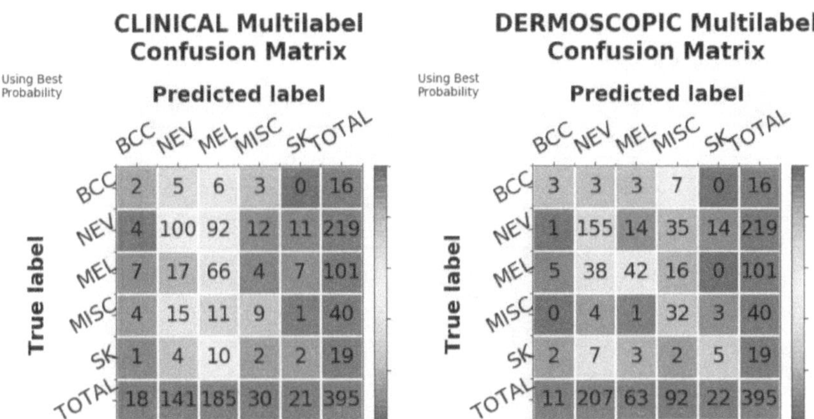

(a) Multilabel confusion matrix for the model trained on clinical images.

(b) Multilabel confusion matrix for the model trained on dermoscopic images.

Figure 5.11: Multilabel confusion matrices for the models of the third experiment.

Table 5.4 contains the metric scores of this experiment, as well as the second and third experiment for comparison. The model trained on clinical images (CImgMd_CF_TransfL7pts) outperforms the class-fusion model (CImgMd_CF), as is indicated by the higher global accuracy and higher average metric scores. The model did not obtain as high performance as in the class-fusion model on the BCC class, but it did improve over the results from multitasking (res3) and baseline (res1) models. All of the classes saw an improvement in their metric scores, with the improvement on the MEL class seeming the largest, contributing the most for the higher global accuracy and higher average metric scores.

The model trained on dermoscopic images (DImgMd_CF_TransfL7pts) improved as well, but not as much as the CImgMd_CF_TransfL7pts. Its global accuracy increased, with the average SPC, F1 and AUROC increasing as well, only the average SEN falls short of the DImg_MT7pts. The BCC class improves over the class-fusion model (DImgMd_CF) due to a higher F1-score, this is due to a higher SPC score, as it does have a lower SEN and AUROC score. Different from the CImgMd_CF_TransfL7pts, the model did not improve its performance on all of the classes, as the performance over MEL and SK was worse than the DImg_MT7pts, with the performance over the SK class being worse than the DImgMd_CF. Despite this, the global accuracy is higher due to a higher performance in the NEV class, obtaining better results in most metric scores, together with the MISC class.

Figure 5.12 shows the multitlabel confusion matrix for the models of the fourth experiments. The matrices show that in the BCC class, with a similar number of predictions to the Img_MT7pts (Figure 5.11), there was an increase in the number of true positives. The CImgMd_CF_TransfL7pts increased both the number of predictions and the true pos-

Table 5.4: Test metric scores for the ImgMd_CF_TransfL7pts (exp4) experiment and its closest comparisons, ImgMd_CF (exp2) and Img_MT7pts (exp3).

EXP		CImgMd_CF_TransfL7pts					DImgMd_CF_TransfL7pts				
		ACC	SEN	SPC	F1	AUROC	ACC	SEN	SPC	F1	AUROC
4	BCC		0.31	0.97	0.29	0.74		0.31	**0.98**	**0.36**	0.78
	NEV		0.6	0.73	0.66	0.73		**0.81**	0.65	**0.78**	**0.81**
	MEL	0.54	0.57	**0.76**	**0.5**	**0.69**	0.64	0.41	0.92	0.5	0.7
	MISC		0.43	0.91	0.38	0.77		0.68	**0.89**	**0.51**	**0.89**
	SK		0.16	0.96	0.17	0.56		0.16	0.97	0.18	0.82
	AVG		**0.414**	**0.866**	**0.4**	**0.698**		0.474	**0.882**	**0.466**	**0.8**
EXP		CImgMd_CF					DImgMd_CF				
2	BCC		**0.38**	0.96	**0.31**	0.86		**0.38**	0.96	0.32	**0.87**
	NEV		0.51	0.76	0.6	0.71		0.42	**0.80**	0.53	0.68
	MEL	0.46	0.46	0.71	0.39	0.6	0.45	0.42	0.86	0.45	0.66
	MISC		0.35	0.86	0.27	0.67		**0.85**	0.67	0.36	0.83
	SK		0.16	0.95	0.15	0.61		**0.26**	**0.98**	**0.32**	0.82
	AVG		0.372	0.848	0.344	0.69		0.466	0.854	0.396	0.772
EXP		CImg_MT7pts					DImg_MT7pts				
3	BCC		0.13	0.96	0.12	0.64		0.19	0.98	0.22	0.74
	NEV		0.46	0.77	0.56	0.69		0.71	0.7	0.73	0.79
	MEL	0.45	0.65	0.60	0.46	0.68	0.6	**0.42**	**0.93**	**0.51**	**0.76**
	MISC		0.23	0.94	0.26	0.7		0.8	0.83	0.48	0.87
	SK		0.11	0.95	0.1	0.56		0.26	0.95	0.24	0.82
	AVG		0.316	0.844	0.3	0.654		**0.476**	0.878	0.436	0.796

itives of NEV and MISC classes, with the MEL class having the opposite effect. The SK class had a decrease in the number of predictions and an increase in the number of true positives. The DImgMd_CF_TransfL7pts had the same occurrence in the NEV class as the CImgMd_CF_TransfL7pts, increasing the number of predictions and true positives, in comparison with the DImg_MT7pts. MEL reached similar numbers as the DImg_MT7pts, but with one less true positive and one more prediction. MISC and SK classes both had lower numbers of true positives and predictions, however MISC ended up lowering the number of predictions in a higher rate than the true positives.

Transferring the learned knowledge from the third experiment improved the class-fusion. It allowed the models to keep their higher performance in the larger classes, while also increasing their performance in the BCC class. The model trained on dermoscopic images benefited the most from this setup, as straight class-fusion with metadata impacted heavily its performance on the larger classes, lowering the global accuracy. It is worth mentioning that the effects of class-fusing with metadata, the higher performance in the BCC class, are not present in their totality. This is observed in the lower performance over the BCC class when compared with the

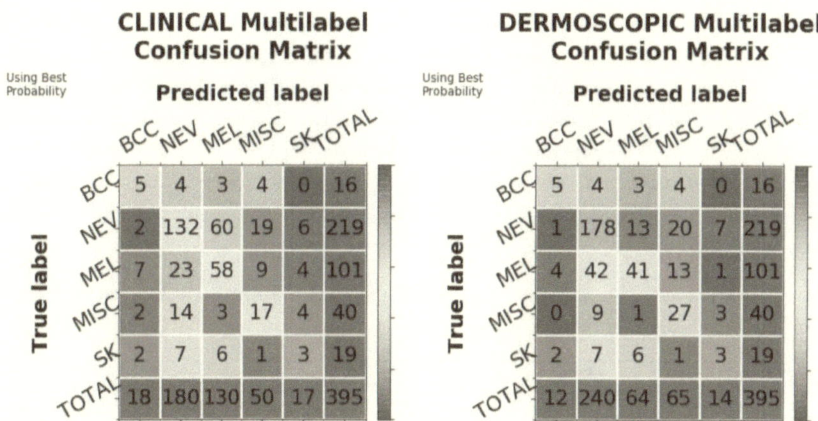

(a) Multilabel confusion matrix for the model trained on clinical images.

(b) Multilabel confusion matrix for the model trained on dermoscopic images.

Figure 5.12: Multilabel confusion matrices for the models of the fourth experiment.

ImgMT_CF.

5.6 Img_MTMd (exp5)

Utilizing the model explained in Subsection exp5, multitasking is performed with metadata instead of the 7-points.

The model trained with clinical images (CImg_MTMd) obtained the metric scores seen in Table 5.5. Global accuracy and average metric scores were higher than the CImg_MT7pts, with only the average SEN and AUROC being lower compared to those of the CImg. This is due to the improvement over all classes except the SK class, comparing to the CImg. The largest increase happens in the BCC class, where nearly all scores increased. The performance over the NEV class is the next to increase the most, having an increase in SEN and F1. There is a slight increase on the performances over the MEL and MISC classes. As both have only an increase of 0.01 in both F1 and AUROC over the CImg, which means that the performance of the MEL class did not surpass that of the CImg_MT7pts. The performance over the SK class is slightly lower than that of the CImg_MT7pts, with its SEN score being one of the reasons for the lower average SEN than that of CImg.

The model trained with dermoscopic images, although performing better than the model trained on clinical images (CImg_MTMd), obtained lower metric scores than the other models trained on dermoscopic images. It obtained lower global accuracy, as well as lower average SEN, SPC, F1 and AUROC. Like the CImg_MTMd, the performance over the BCC class improved, however to a lower degree, as there was only an increase of 0.01 in SPC and 0.02 in F1 from the DImg. The model performed worse over the NEV, MEL and SK classes, when compared with the DImg_MT7pts. The performance over the NEV class was only slightly worse, with a decrease of 0.01 F1-score. The performance over the SK class, althou similar to the DImg, is worse than the DImg_MT7pts. The worst performance is over the MEL class, losing 0.06 F1-score and 0.13 SEN from the DImg. Lastly there is the MISC class, that, despite different SEN and SPC values, obtains the same F1-score, albeit with a lower AUROC as the DImg, indicating a similar performance.

Table 5.5: Test metric scores for the Img_MTMd (exp5) experiment and its closest comparisons, Img (exp1) and Img_MT7pts (exp3).

EXP		CImg_MTMd					DImg_MTMd				
		ACC	SEN	SPC	F1	AUROC	ACC	SEN	SPC	F1	AUROC
	BCC		**0.31**	**0.94**	**0.23**	0.68		**0.31**	0.97	**0.3**	0.81
	NEV		**0.5**	0.78	**0.6**	0.71		0.69	0.71	0.72	0.79
5	MEL	0.47	0.55	0.67	0.44	0.67	0.57	0.37	0.89	0.44	0.74
	MISC		**0.35**	0.93	**0.35**	**0.74**		0.75	0.85	**0.49**	0.83
	SK		0.11	0.93	0.09	0.61		0.16	0.94	0.14	0.82
	AVG		0.364	**0.85**	**0.342**	0.682		0.456	0.872	0.418	0.798

EXP		CImg					DImg				
	BCC		0.25	0.93	0.18	**0.7**		0.31	0.96	**0.28**	0.82
	NEV		0.47	0.79	0.57	0.72		0.67	0.78	0.73	0.79
1	MEL	0.44	0.5	0.71	0.43	0.66	0.59	**0.50**	0.83	**0.51**	0.73
	MISC		0.33	**0.94**	0.34	0.73		0.68	0.88	0.49	**0.87**
	SK		**0.32**	0.86	**0.16**	0.61		0.16	0.96	0.16	0.82
	AVG		**0.374**	0.846	0.336	**0.684**		0.464	**0.882**	0.434	**0.806**

EXP		CImg_MT7pts					DImg_MT7pts				
	BCC		0.13	0.96	0.12	0.64		0.19	0.98	0.22	0.74
	NEV		0.46	0.77	0.56	0.69		0.71	0.7	**0.73**	0.79
3	MEL	0.45	**0.65**	0.60	**0.46**	**0.68**	0.6	0.42	0.93	0.51	0.76
	MISC		0.23	0.94	0.26	0.7		0.8	0.83	0.48	0.87
	SK		0.11	0.95	0.1	0.56		**0.26**	0.95	**0.24**	0.82
	AVG		0.316	0.844	0.3	0.654		**0.476**	0.878	**0.436**	0.796

Figure 5.11 shows the multitlabel confusion matrix for the models of the third experiment. Both matrices show the same number of true positives for the BCC class, however the CImg_MTMd has 10 more predictions than the DImg_MTMd. Comparing with CImg (Figure 5.9a) the CImg_MTMd increases the true positives while reducing the predictions. The model predicts more samples as NEV, MEL and MISC, however the majority of the new predictions in MEL are not correctly classified. The model does the oposite for the SK class, decreasing both the number of predictions and true positives. The DImg_MTMd, in comparison with the DImg (Figure 5.9a) lowers the number of predictions on the BCC, MEL and SK. The

BCC class maintains the same true positives, while MEL and SK have a large drop in the number of true positives. the model predicts more samples in the NEV and MISC classes, however much of these new predictions were misclassified samples.

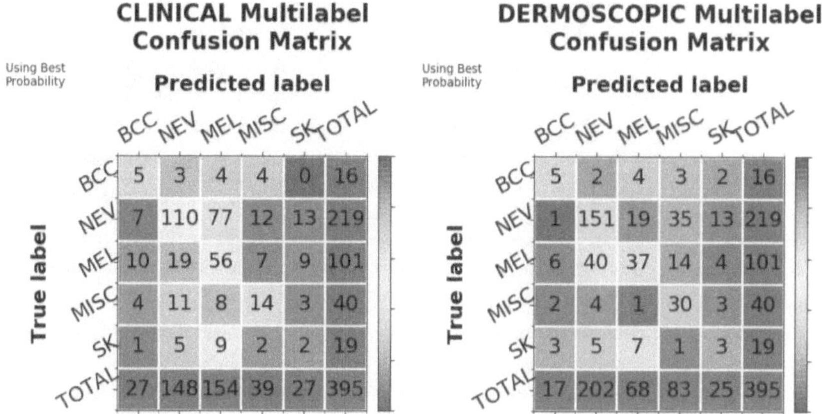

(a) Multilabel confusion matrix for the model trained on clinical images.

(b) Multilabel confusion matrix for the model trained on dermoscopic images.

Figure 5.13: Multilabel confusion matrices for the models of the fifth experiment.

Multitasking with metadata improved the performance of the CImg_MTMd by improving the performance over the BCC class while not impacting negatively the other classes. DImg_MTMd saw an increase in performance over the BCC class as well, but it did not improve much over what the model already knew, as well as negatively impacting the other classes, especially the MEL class. The common points are the improvement of the BCC class and the worsening of the SK class, however these improvements are limited to the information present in the images, as, although the DImg_MTMd improved its performance of the BCC class, it did not improve to near the same level as the CImg_MTMd. A reason for this is that the CImg_MTMd was not extracting as much information from the clinical images as it could to improve the performance over the BCC class, while the DImg_MTMd was already extracting as much information as it could from the dermoscopic images to support its performance over the BCC class.

5.7 ImgMd_CF_TransfLMd (exp6)

Transfer learning the knowledge (weights and bias) obtained by multitasking the metadata, following the model outlined in Subsection exp6, improved upon the results of class-fusion, as can be seen in the metric scores of Table 5.6.

The model trained on clinical images (CImgMd_CF_TransfLMd) obtained slightly lower results compared to the results from the other transfer learning experiment (res4). It managed to obtain similar global accuracy, similar average SPC and AUROC, but the average SEN and F1 were lower than those of CImgMd_CF_TransfL7pts. The performance over the BCC class, the class that benefits the most from the metadata, did improve over the previous experiment, CImg_MTMd, by improving the SPC, F1 and AUROC, but did not reach as high performance as the CImgMd_CF_TransfL7pts or the CImgMd_CF. The performance over the NEV class was the best of all these experiments, with the highest SEN and F1 for any model trained on clinical images. the performance over MEL and SK both improved compared to the CImg_MTMd and CImgMd_CF, but MEL did not surpass CImgMd_CF_TransfL7pts while SK has similar results. MISC remained relatively unchanged, with small changes to SEN and SPC, but the same F1 as the CImg_MTMd, which is lower than the one from the CImgMd_CF_TransfL7pts.

The model trained on dermoscopic images (DImgMd_CF_TransfLMd), much like the clinical version, improved upon the previous experiment (DImg_MTMd), but fell short of the DImgMd_CF_TransfL7pts. The difference is it obtaining the highest average SEN of the dermoscopic models, due to the high SEN of the MISC and SK classes. Although these two classes have high SEN, only the performance over the SK class was better than the other models, with MISC reaching the same 0.49 F1 as the DImg_MTMd, which is above the 0.36 of the DImgMd_CF, but below the 0.51 from the DImgMd_CF_TransfL7pts. There is an improvement in the performance over both NEV and MEL over the DImg_MTMd and DImgMd_CF, but fall short of the performance from DImgMd_CF_TransfL7pts. The performance over the BCC class is strange, as it is worse than all of the other models, when it was expected to be at the same level or better. It obtained a lower SEN score, with the SPC increasing by 0.01. This is too small of an increase in SPC to balance the lower SEN score, as is shown by the lower F1-score of 0.22. Even DImgMd_CF_TransfL7pts has the same SPC with a higher SEN score.

Figure 5.14 shows the multitlabel confusion matrix for the models of the sixth experiment. The CImgMd_CF_TransfLMd improves slightly on the BCC class, maintaining the number of true positives and decreasing the predictions when comparing with the CImg_MTMd (Figure 5.13a). There is an improvement in the SK class by increasing the number of true positives with less predictions, while NEV and MISC have an increase of predictions, some of which are true positives (+29 NEV and +1 MISC). MEL sees a large reduction on the predictions, of which only 3 were true positives.

DImgMd_CF_TransfLMd goes through similar changes as the CImgMd_CF_TransfLMd. NEV and MISC receiving more predictions than the DImg_MTMd (Figure 5.13b), of which some were true positives (+4 NEV and +4 MISC), SK increasing the number of correctly classified samples by 4 while reducing the number of predictions by 2 and MEL having a small reduction (-13) in the number of predictions, where only 1 was a true positive. The difference occurs in the BCC class, as there is a reduction on the number of predictions, two of which were true positives.

Transferring the learned knowledge obtained by multitasking the metadata did improve the performance of the models when they handled both images and metadata. Like the other transfer learning experiment, ImgMd_CF_TransfL7pts (exp4), the large negative impacts on the performance of the larger classes were reduced but the full improvement to the performance

Table 5.6: Test metric scores for the ImgMd_CF_TransfLMd (exp6) experiment and its closest comparisons, ImgMd_CF (exp2), ImgMd_CF_TransfL7pts (exp4) and Img_MTMd (exp5).

EXP		CImgMd_CF_TransfLMd					DImgMd_CF_TransfLMd				
		ACC	SEN	SPC	F1	AUROC	ACC	SEN	SPC	F1	AUROC
6	BCC		0.31	0.96	0.26	0.77		0.19	0.98	0.22	0.76
	NEV		**0.63**	0.72	**0.68**	0.73		0.71	0.7	0.73	0.77
	MEL	0.54	0.52	**0.77**	0.48	0.67	0.59	0.36	**0.94**	0.46	0.71
	MISC		0.38	0.91	0.35	0.75		**0.85**	0.82	0.49	0.84
	SK		0.16	**0.97**	0.17	0.56		**0.37**	0.96	**0.33**	0.85
	AVG		0.4	**0.866**	0.388	**0.696**		**0.496**	0.88	0.446	0.786

EXP		CImgMd_CF					DImgMd_CF				
		ACC	SEN	SPC	F1	AUROC	ACC	SEN	SPC	F1	AUROC
2	BCC		**0.38**	0.96	**0.31**	0.86		0.38	0.96	0.32	**0.87**
	NEV		0.51	0.76	0.6	0.71		0.42	0.80	0.53	0.68
	MEL	0.46	0.46	0.71	0.39	0.6	0.45	**0.42**	0.86	0.45	0.66
	MISC		0.35	0.86	0.27	0.67		0.85	0.67	0.36	0.83
	SK		0.16	0.95	0.15	0.61		0.26	0.98	0.32	0.82
	AVG		0.372	0.848	0.344	0.69		0.466	0.854	0.396	0.772

EXP		CImgMd_CF_TransfL7pts					DImgMd_CF_TransfL7pts				
		ACC	SEN	SPC	F1	AUROC	ACC	SEN	SPC	F1	AUROC
4	BCC		0.31	**0.97**	0.29	0.74		0.31	**0.98**	**0.36**	0.78
	NEV		0.6	0.73	0.66	0.73		**0.81**	0.65	**0.78**	0.81
	MEL	0.54	**0.57**	0.76	**0.5**	0.69	**0.64**	0.41	0.92	**0.5**	0.7
	MISC		**0.43**	0.91	**0.38**	0.77		0.68	0.89	**0.51**	0.89
	SK		0.16	0.96	0.17	0.56		0.16	0.97	0.18	0.82
	AVG		**0.414**	0.866	**0.4**	0.698		0.474	**0.882**	**0.466**	**0.8**

EXP		CImg_MTMd					DImg_MTMd				
		ACC	SEN	SPC	F1	AUROC	ACC	SEN	SPC	F1	AUROC
5	BCC		0.31	0.94	0.23	0.68		0.31	0.97	0.3	0.81
	NEV		0.5	0.78	0.6	0.71		0.69	0.71	0.72	0.79
	MEL	0.47	0.55	0.67	0.44	0.67	0.57	0.37	0.89	0.44	0.74
	MISC		0.35	0.93	0.35	0.74		0.75	0.85	0.49	0.83
	SK		0.11	0.93	0.09	0.61		0.16	0.94	0.14	0.82
	AVG		0.364	0.85	0.342	0.682		0.456	0.872	0.418	0.798

over the BCC class was not achieved. Overall this improves the model, making it more well rounded in its performance over the various classes, rather than being biased in favor of one or another class due to either a higher number of samples, or a biased modality. However the results obtained by the ImgMd_CF_TransfL7pts were better, especially with the dermoscopic images.

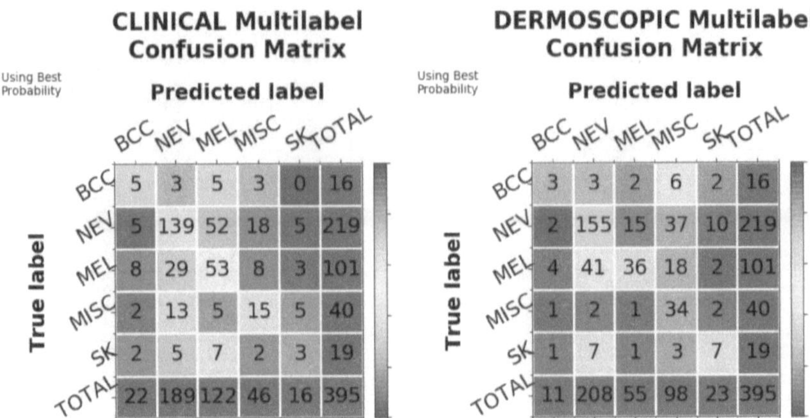

(a) Multilabel confusion matrix for the model trained on clinical images.

(b) Multilabel confusion matrix for the model trained on dermoscopic images.

Figure 5.14: Multilabel confusion matrices for the models of the sixth experiment.

5.8 ImgMd_FF (exp7)

Feature-fusion is used to join the metadata with the images, utilizing the model outlaid in Subsection exp7. This approach shows better average metric scores than if class-fusion were utilised. A reason for this is seen in the metric scores in Table 5.7, where there is a better performance over NEV from both models, either trained on clinical images or dermoscopic images. Despite the better performance over NEV though, the performance over the BCC class was not as high as the class-fusion models.

In the model trained on clinical images (CImgMd_FF) the performance over the BCC class does improve, but at a much reduced rate than with class-fusion (CImgMd_CF). Rather, the performance over every class sees an improvement, even if small. Were the results of the CImgMd_CF in MEL, MISC and SK were lower than the baseline (CImg), with a large increase of the results on the BCC class, the CImgMd_FF increases the performance over every class, surpassing the CImg, and CImgMd_CF in all but the BCC class.

The performance from the model trained on dermoscopic images (DImgMd_FF) was different. Although obtaining slightly higher global accuracy and average metrics than the dermoscopic baseline (DImg), the model only performs better for the NEV and SK classes, with the SK class seeing lower results than the class-fusion model (DImgMd_CF). The performance for the MISC class is better than the DImgMd_CF, but slightly lower than the DImg. The performance over the MEL class was similar to that of the DImgMd_CF, but with different SEN and SPC scores. It did manage to obtain an higher AUROC score (0.71), but the results obtained are still lower than the DImg. Lastly, the performance over the BCC class decreases when compared to the DImg. This result was unexpected, as previous inclusions of metadata lead to an increase of the performance over the BCC class. This can be explained by the higher detail from the dermoscopic images leading to an already high performance over the BCC class. In this case, the model has difficulty fusing the information regarding the BCC class from the metadata and from the dermoscopic images. This results in the model performing worse when it has more control over the feature selection, which is what feature-fusion provides.

Table 5.7: Test metric scores for the ImgMd_FF (exp7) experiment and its closest comparisons, Img (exp1) and ImgMd_CF (exp2).

EXP		CImgMd_FF					DImgMd_FF				
		ACC	SEN	SPC	F1	AUROC	ACC	SEN	SPC	F1	AUROC
7	BCC		0.25	0.96	0.23	0.8		0.25	**0.97**	0.26	0.88
	NEV		**0.59**	0.76	**0.66**	0.76		**0.73**	0.78	**0.76**	0.82
	MEL	0.52	**0.54**	0.71	**0.46**	0.69	0.6	0.38	**0.9**	0.45	0.71
	MISC		**0.38**	0.92	**0.36**	0.75		0.8	0.81	0.46	0.86
	SK		0.21	0.95	**0.2**	0.71		0.26	0.97	0.29	0.8
	AVG		**0.394**	**0.86**	**0.382**	**0.742**		**0.484**	**0.886**	**0.444**	**0.814**
EXP		CImg					DImg				
1	BCC		0.25	0.93	0.18	0.7		0.31	0.96	0.28	0.82
	NEV		0.47	0.79	0.57	0.72		0.67	0.78	0.73	0.79
	MEL	0.44	0.5	0.71	0.43	0.66	0.59	**0.50**	0.83	**0.51**	0.73
	MISC		0.33	**0.94**	0.34	0.73		0.68	**0.88**	**0.49**	0.87
	SK		**0.32**	0.86	0.16	0.61		0.16	0.96	0.16	0.82
	AVG		0.374	0.846	0.336	0.684		0.464	0.882	0.434	0.806
EXP		CImgMd_CF					DImgMd_CF				
2	BCC		**0.38**	0.96	**0.31**	0.86		**0.38**	0.96	**0.32**	0.87
	NEV		0.51	0.76	0.6	0.71		0.42	0.80	0.53	0.68
	MEL	0.46	0.46	0.71	0.39	0.6	0.45	0.42	0.86	0.45	0.66
	MISC		0.35	0.86	0.27	0.67		**0.85**	0.67	0.36	0.83
	SK		0.16	0.95	0.15	0.61		0.26	**0.98**	**0.32**	0.82
	AVG		0.372	0.848	0.344	0.69		0.466	0.854	0.396	0.772

Figure 5.15 shows the multilabel confusion matrices for the seventh experiment, here is clearly seen that both matrices have high numbers of SK samples predicted as MEL. Comparing the matrices from the CImgMd_FF, Figure 5.15a, and the CImgMd_CF, shows an increase in both the total predictions and true positives of NEV and MEL, justifying the higher metric scores from the table. There is a decrease of total predictions on MISC, from 64, with a small increase in the true positives, from 14. The SK class is interesting, as it does not change the total predictions, but increases the true positives by 1. The DImgMd_FF matrix, Figure 5.15b, shows the MEL class with similar proportion of true positives to total predictions as the DImgMd_CF. MISC, comparing with DImgMd_CF, has 50 less total predictions, 2 of which were true positives. The SK class obtains 3 more total predictions, but maintains the same number of true positives (5).

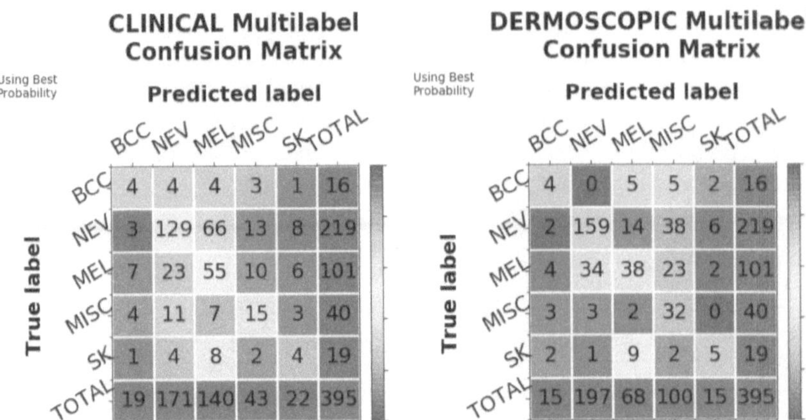

(a) Multilabel confusion matrix for the model trained on clinical images.

(b) Multilabel confusion matrix for the model trained on dermoscopic images.

Figure 5.15: Multilabel confusion matrices for the models of the seventh experiment.

Similar to the class-fusion experiment, feature fusion had a similar impact over the baseline. For clinical images, it provides general improvements for all classes, class-fusion did this to a degree, but focused more on the BCC class. For dermoscopic images, feature-fusion brought an increase for the NEV and SK class, reducing the cost of this on the other classes. This is in some opposition to what class-fusion did, as class-fusion managed to further increase the performance of the BCC and SK classes, by reducing the performance over the NEV and MISC classes. MEL performed similarly in both dermoscopic fusions. Feature-fusion produced better global accuracy and better average metric scores than class-fusion, as well as it producing a more balanced outcome, reducing the bias in favor of the BCC class that class-fusion applied. As such, it seems that feature-fusion is better at fusing modalities by providing a more balanced performance.

5.9 ImgMd_FF_MT7pts (exp8)

The multitasking of the 7-points in the feature-fusion of image and metadata, with the model from Subsection exp8, revealed an overall better results than either class-fusion or feature-fusion, as can be seen on Table 5.8.

For the model trained on clinical images (CImgMd_FF_MT7pts), the global accuracy, as well as the average metric scores improved over the class-fusion (CImgMd_CF) and feature-fusion (ImgMd_FF). There is an increase in the performance for every class over the CImgMd_FF, with the performance on the BCC class being similar to that of CImgMd_CF, as it obtained similar F1 and AUROC scores despite having different SEN and SPC scores.

For the model trained on dermoscopic images (DImgMd_FF_MT7pts), there is an increase in the global accuracy, as well as the average scores for SEN and F1, but the average metric scores for the SPC and AUROC reduce by 0.004 and 0.024 respectively from the best scores obtained by DImgMd_FF. This model obtained the best performance over the BCC class, with the highest SPC and F1-score, but lower AUROC than fusion without multitasking. The performance over the NEV class lowered slightly, comparing to the best performance of DImgMd_FF, it did however obtain the highest SEN score. The performance over MISC increased, but remains slightly lower than the DImg (0.48 vs 0.49 F1-score and 0.86 vs 0.87 AUROC). The performance over the MEL class is similar to the other fusion models trained on dermoscopic images, obtaining similar F1-score. This performance is lower than that of the DImg (0.51 F1-score), however the DImgMd_FF_MT7pts acquired the best AUROC score (0.75 vs 0.73 DImg) and SPC score (0.93 vs 0.83 DImg). The results show the same SEN score for the SK class across the models, with varying scores for the SPC, F1 and AUROC. The DImgMd_FF_MT7pts reduced the F1-score of the SK class by 0.01 from the lowest (0.29 DImgMd_FF), while obtaining the lowest AUROC score. This is still a better performance than the DImg over the SK class.

Table 5.8: Test metric scores for the ImgMd_FF_MT7pts (exp8) experiment and its closest comparisons, ImgMd_CF (exp2) and ImgMd_FF (exp7).

EXP		CImgMd_FF_MT7pts					DImgMd_FF_MT7pts				
		ACC	SEN	SPC	F1	AUROC	ACC	SEN	SPC	F1	AUROC
	BCC		0.31	**0.97**	**0.31**	0.86		0.38	**0.98**	**0.39**	0.81
	NEV		**0.61**	**0.8**	**0.69**	0.77		**0.76**	0.68	0.75	0.8
8	MEL	0.56	**0.61**	0.7	**0.49**	0.68	0.61	0.35	**0.93**	0.45	**0.75**
	MISC		**0.4**	**0.95**	**0.44**	0.79		0.75	**0.85**	**0.48**	0.86
	SK		**0.32**	0.94	**0.26**	0.71		0.26	0.97	0.28	0.73
	AVG		**0.45**	**0.872**	**0.438**	**0.762**		**0.5**	0.882	**0.47**	0.79
EXP		CImgMd_CF					DImgMd_CF				
	BCC		**0.38**	0.96	0.31	0.86		0.38	0.96	0.32	0.87
	NEV		0.51	0.76	0.6	0.71		0.42	**0.80**	0.53	0.68
2	MEL	0.46	**0.46**	0.71	0.39	0.6	0.45	0.42	0.86	0.45	0.66
	MISC		0.35	0.86	0.27	0.67		**0.85**	0.67	0.36	0.83
	SK		0.16	0.95	0.15	0.61		0.26	**0.98**	**0.32**	0.82
	AVG		0.372	0.848	0.344	0.69		0.466	0.854	0.396	0.772
EXP		CImgMd_FF					DImgMd_FF				
	BCC		0.25	0.96	0.23	0.8		0.25	0.97	0.26	0.88
	NEV		0.59	0.76	0.66	0.76		0.73	0.78	**0.76**	0.82
7	MEL	0.52	0.54	0.71	0.46	0.69	0.6	0.38	0.9	0.45	0.71
	MISC		0.38	0.92	0.36	0.75		0.8	0.81	0.46	0.86
	SK		0.21	0.95	0.2	0.71		0.26	0.97	0.29	0.8
	AVG		0.394	0.86	0.382	0.742		0.484	**0.886**	0.444	**0.814**

Figure 5.16 shows the multilabel confusion matrices for the eighth experiment. In these

experiments, the improvement of the BCC class is noticeable, with an increase in the correctly classified samples and lower number of predictions, compared with the baseline (Figure 5.9) and feature-fusion (Figure 5.15), with the CImgMd_CL (Figure 5.10a) having more correctly classified samples, but more predictions as well. The CImgMd_FF_MT7pts shows clear improvement on the NEV and MISC classes, with lower number of predictions and a higher number of correctly classified samples. There is an increase in the number of predictions for the MEL and SK some of which are correctly classified, resulting in a general increase in the accuracy of those classes. The DImgMd_FF_MT7pts has a large increase in the number of predictions of the NEV class, with only a small portion of these being correctly classified, resulting in a lower accuracy for the class. While there is a decrease of the number of predictions on both the MEL and MISC classes, in the case of MEL, some of those were correctly classified, resulting in similar accuracy with the other models. As with the MISC class, only a small number of the removed predictions were correctly classified, resulting in an increase in the accuracy of the class. Lastly, the model loses performance on the SK class by having more predictions than were misclassified samples.

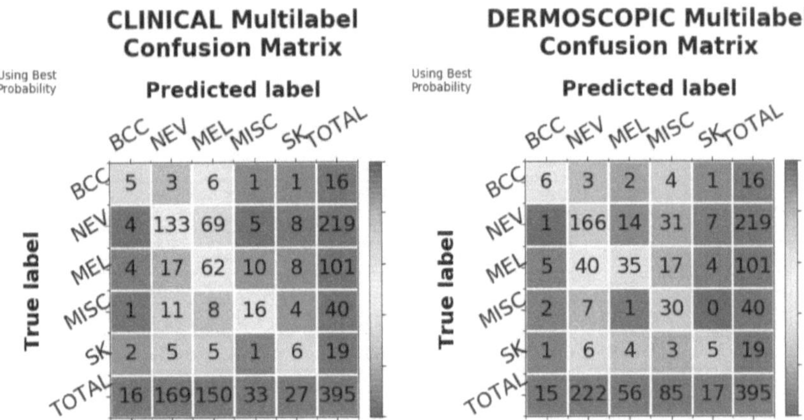

(a) Multilabel confusion matrix for the model trained on clinical images.

(b) Multilabel confusion matrix for the model trained on dermoscopic images.

Figure 5.16: Multilabel confusion matrices for the models of the eighth experiment.

Class-fusion (exp2) brings a large increase to the performance on the BCC class in both types of images, with a reduced performance on the other classes. Feature-fusion (exp7) improves the performance of BCC for the clinical images and NEV and SK for dermoscopic images, while reducing the negative impact on the large classes. Multitasking the 7-points with the feature-fusion provides another general improvement for the models trained on clinical images, while providing some benefits to models trained on dermoscopic images. The multitasking in the models trained on dermoscopic images seems to facilitate the fusion of the dermoscopic images with the metadata, as there is further improvement to the performance over the BCC class. This can be due to the multitasking forcing the model to select better features from both modalities.

As such multitasking the 7-points with the feature-fusion is a good addition to increase the overall performance of the model and extracting more information from the modalities.

5.10   2Img_FF_MT7pts (exp9)

This experiment utilizes the model from the Subsection exp9 where both image types are used to classify the lesions. The images are fused through feature-fusion and there is multitasking of the categories of the 7-points in addition to the lesion classification.

The results obtained by this experiment can be seen on the metric score Table 5.9. A high global accuracy of 0.63 was obtained, however most average metric scores did not surpass those of DImgMd_FF_MT7pts, such as the average SEN, F1 and AUROC. Compared with the models trained on only a type of image, Img_MT7pts, this model has a better performance in the BCC class, obtaining a SEN that rivals that of the CImgMd_FF_MT7pts and DImg of 0.31, however the best performance still belongs to the DImgMd_FF_MT7pts. The model obtains the best metric scores for the MEL class, while the performance on NEV is slightly below that of the DImgMd_CF_TransfL7pts, which has the highest performance in the NEV class. The performance of the model over MISC and SK does not improve, with the performance over MISC being similar to the models trained on dermoscopic images, such as DImg_MT7pts and DImgMd_FF_MT7pts, while the performance over SK is only higher than the CImg_MT7pts, as is reflected by the F1-scores.

Figure 5.17 shows the multilabel confusion matrix and the ROC curves for the ninth experiment, 2Img_FF_MT7pts. There performance over the BCC class is strange as there is an abrupt decrease in performance between the values of 0.4/0.1 to 0.9/0.65 (TPR/FPR). The multilabel confusion matrix (Figure 5.17a) shows a good overall result, with the number of predictions for each class closely resembling the real number of samples of the class. Together, the predictions of the NEV class are more than half correctly classified, MEL has about half of its predictions correctly classified, and MISC has one less then half of its predictions correctly classified. Both BCC and SK received more predictions than the ImgMd_FF_MT7pts (Figure 5.16), but these were misclassifications, with SK even having a lower number of correctly classified samples.

Using solely both image types improves the performance of BCC and MEL over image models and improves NEV over the feature-fusion with multitasking models. The MISC class sees a reduction of its predictions from models trained on dermoscopic images, but maintains the same performance, as is supported by the same F1-score. This indicates that the performance of the other classes improved, reducing the bias the dermoscopic models had to predict more samples as MISC. The performance of the SK class did improve, but not as much as utilizing just the dermoscopic images, or a fusion of images with metadata.

Table 5.9: Test metric scores for the 2Img_FF_MT7pts (exp9) experiment and its closest comparisons, Img_MT7pts (exp3) and ImgMd_FF_MT7pts (exp8).

EXP		2Img_FF_MT7pts									
		ACC	SEN	SPC	F1	AUROC	ACC	SEN	SPC	F1	AUROC
9	BCC		0.31	0.96	0.27	0.64					
	NEV		**0.78**	0.69	**0.77**	0.82					
	MEL	**0.63**	0.5	0.86	**0.52**	**0.77**					
	MISC		0.48	0.94	**0.48**	0.81					
	SK		0.21	0.96	0.21	0.77					
	AVG		0.456	**0.882**	0.45	0.762					

EXP		CImg_MT7pts					DImg_MT7pts				
3	BCC		0.13	0.96	0.12	0.64		0.19	0.98	0.22	0.74
	NEV		0.46	0.77	0.56	0.69		0.71	0.7	0.73	0.79
	MEL	0.45	0.65	0.60	0.46	0.68	0.6	0.42	0.93	0.51	0.76
	MISC		0.23	0.94	0.26	0.7		**0.8**	0.83	**0.48**	0.87
	SK		0.11	0.95	0.1	0.56		0.26	0.95	0.24	0.82
	AVG		0.316	0.844	0.3	0.654		0.476	0.878	0.436	0.796

EXP		CImgMd_FF_MT7pts					DImgMd_FF_MT7pts				
8	BCC		0.31	0.97	0.31	0.86		**0.38**	0.98	**0.39**	0.81
	NEV		0.61	**0.8**	0.69	0.77		0.76	0.68	0.75	0.8
	MEL	0.56	**0.61**	0.7	0.49	0.68	0.61	0.35	**0.93**	0.45	0.75
	MISC		0.4	**0.95**	0.44	0.79		0.75	0.85	**0.48**	0.86
	SK		**0.32**	0.94	0.26	0.71		0.26	**0.97**	**0.28**	0.73
	AVG		0.45	0.872	0.438	0.762		**0.5**	0.882	**0.47**	**0.79**

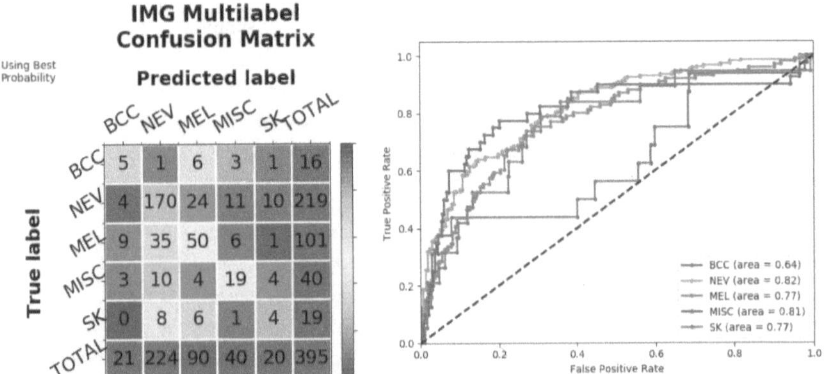

(a) Multilabel confusion matrix for the model trained on both images.

(b) ROC curves for the model trained on both images.

Figure 5.17: Multilabel confusion matrix and ROC curves for the model of the ninth experiment.

5.11   2ImgMd_FF_MT7pts (exp10)

The model explained in Subsection exp10 is used to fuse all of the modalities available, clinical image, dermoscopic image and metadata, through feature-fusion and wile multitasking the categories of the 7-points.

The results are shown in the metric score Table 5.10, these show the highest global accuracy of 0.65, together with an increase in all of the average metric scores, except AUROC. The results for the BCC class are in line with the conclusions obtained about the inclusion of metadata (concluded in res2) and the fusion of both images (concluded in res9), as the performance of the model over the BCC class benefits greatly from these fusions. Only the AUROC metric of the BCC class does not improve at the same pace as the other metrics, as it increases from the ninth experiment (2Img_FF_MT7pts), but it is still lower than the metadata-focused eighth experiment (Img_FF_MT7pts), as well as being the main cause for the lower average AUROC. The performance on NEV steadily improves, while the performance of the MEL class remains similar to that of the DImg_MT7pts, the second best performing model for MEL. the performance on MISC improves, obtaining a high SPC and F1-score, although the AUROC is below the DImg_MT7pts and DImg_FF_MT7pts. The model improves upon the SEN of the SK class, bringing the F1-score to its highest of 0.33, but the AUROC value obtained is similar to those obtained by the Img_FF_MT7pts, not the highest, but not the lowest by far.

Figure 5.18 shows the multilabel confusion matrix and the ROC curves for the tenth experiment. The multilabel confusion matrix seen in the Figure 5.18a has a higher number of correctly classified samples for most classes, when comparing with the ninth experiment, only the MEL class a lesser number. The model reduces the number of predictions for the BCC, MEL and SK classes, these being instead predicted as either NEV or MISC. Seeing as the MEL class has fewer true positives and lower predictions, it is concluded that the resulting accuracy is an improvement, as the majority of the removed predictions were misclassified samples.

The ROC curves, see Figure 5.18b, shows that there are certain points where the model sudenly performs worse on the SK, BCC and MEL classes, specifically, their performance worsens at higher TP/FP rates. This is the reason for the lower AUROC.

Although models trained on dermoscopic images produces better results for some classes, fusion with clinical images provides a general improvement to the results of every class, as can be seen by this (exp10) and the ninth experiment (exp9). The inclusion of Metadata with both images increased the results of the BCC class, while the usage of both images prevented the biasing of the model towards the BCC class.

Table 5.10: Test metric scores for the 2ImgMd_FF_MT7pts (exp10) experiment and its closest comparisons, Img_MT7pts (exp3), ImgMd_FF_MT7pts (exp8) and 2Img_FF_MT7pts (exp9).

EXP		2ImgMd_FF_MT7pts									
		ACC	SEN	SPC	F1	AUROC	ACC	SEN	SPC	F1	AUROC
10	BCC	0.65	**0.44**	0.97	**0.41**	0.73					
	NEV		**0.81**	0.68	**0.78**	**0.84**					
	MEL		0.45	0.89	0.51	0.75					
	MISC		0.58	**0.92**	**0.51**	0.84					
	SK		**0.32**	**0.97**	**0.33**	0.7					
	AVG		**0.52**	**0.886**	**0.508**	0.772					
EXP		CImg_MT7pts					DImg_MT7pts				
3	BCC	0.45	0.13	0.96	0.12	0.64	0.6	0.19	0.98	0.22	0.74
	NEV		0.46	0.77	0.56	0.69		0.71	0.7	0.73	0.79
	MEL		**0.65**	0.60	0.46	0.68		0.42	**0.93**	0.51	0.76
	MISC		0.23	0.94	0.26	0.7		**0.8**	0.83	0.48	**0.87**
	SK		0.11	0.95	0.1	0.56		0.26	0.95	0.24	**0.82**
	AVG		0.316	0.844	0.3	0.654		0.476	0.878	0.436	**0.796**
EXP		CImgMd_FF_MT7pts					DImgMd_FF_MT7pts				
8	BCC	0.56	0.31	0.97	0.31	**0.86**	0.61	0.38	0.98	0.39	0.81
	NEV		0.61	**0.8**	0.69	0.77		0.76	0.68	0.75	0.8
	MEL		0.61	0.7	0.49	0.68		0.35	0.93	0.45	0.75
	MISC		0.4	0.95	0.44	0.79		0.75	0.85	0.48	0.86
	SK		0.32	0.94	0.26	0.71		0.26	0.97	0.28	0.73
	AVG		0.45	0.872	0.438	0.762		0.5	0.882	0.47	0.79
EXP		2Img_FF_MT7pts									
9	BCC	0.63	0.31	0.96	0.27	0.64					
	NEV		0.78	0.69	0.77	0.82					
	MEL		0.5	0.86	**0.52**	**0.77**					
	MISC		0.48	0.94	0.48	0.81					
	SK		0.21	0.96	0.21	0.77					
	AVG		0.456	0.882	0.45	0.762					

5.12 2ImgMd_CombFF_MT7pts (exp11)

In the eleventh experiment, several combinations of modalities are performed in the same model (2ImgMd_CombFF_MT7pts). Effectively, the third, Img_MT7pts, eight, ImgMd_FF_MT7pts, and tenth, 2ImgMd_FF_MT7pts, experiments are performed in a single model, following the structure explained in Subsection exp11. The results are show and discussed in the following subsections: Single image (res11i), Single image and Metadata (res11im) and Clinical image, Dermoscopic images and Metadata (res11cdm). This division facilitates the presentation and

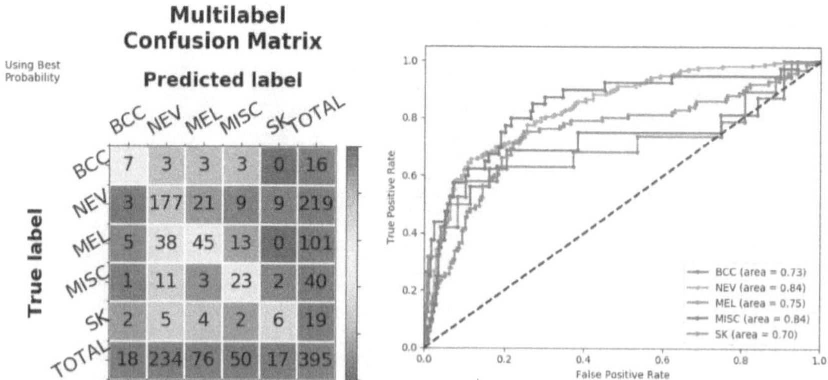

(a) Multilabel confusion matrix for the model (b) ROC curves for the model trained on all modalities. trained on all modalities.

Figure 5.18: Multilabel confusion matrix and ROC curves for the model of the tenth experiment.

discussion of the relevant results for each combination. As the names of the subsections imply, the first Subsection res11i contains the results for the combinations made of solely clinical or dermoscopic images, alongside the results from the third experiment. The second Subsection res11im shows the results for the combinations made of clinical images and metadata or dermoscopic images and metadata, alongside the results from the eight experiment. Lastly, the third Subsection res11cdm shows the results for the combination of all modalities, clinical images, dermoscopic images and metadata, alongside the results from the tenth experiment.

5.12.1 Single image

The single image combinations from the 2ImgMd_CombFF_MT7pts obtained subtle differences in the results, as can be observed in the metric score Table 5.11.

The clinical image combination of the 2ImgMd_CombFF_MT7pts obtained lower global accuracy, but higher average SEN, F1 and AUROC. The reason for the higher average SEN is the SEN scores from the BCC and SK classes, where the model obtained a higher value than CImg_MT7pts. The lower global accuracy comes from the lower performance on the MEL class and equal performance of the NEV class, since these classes have a larger number of samples. Lastly, there is a slight increase in the SEN and F1-score of the MISC class.

The dermoscopic image combination of the 2ImgMd_CombFF_MT7pts obtained lower global accuracy and lower average SEN, F1-score and AUROC, with the average SPC being the same as DImg_MT7pts. Different from the clinical variant, the performances on the BCC and the NEV classes improves. However the improvement in the performance of the NEV class is not high enough to compensate for the lower performance in the MEL, MISC and SK classes, explaining the lower global accuracy and lower average metrics.

Table 5.11: Test metric scores for the 2ImgMd_CombFF_MT7pts (Single image) (exp11) experiment and its equivalent, Img_MT7pts (exp3).

EXP		2ImgMd_CombFF_MT7pts (CImg)					2ImgMd_CombFF_MT7pts (DImg)				
		ACC	SEN	SPC	F1	AUROC	ACC	SEN	SPC	F1	AUROC
11	BCC		**0.19**	0.95	**0.16**	0.73		**0.25**	0.97	**0.25**	0.72
	NEV		0.46	0.77	0.56	0.69		0.71	**0.73**	**0.74**	0.79
	MEL	0.44	0.55	**0.67**	0.44	0.65	0.58	0.37	0.92	0.46	0.67
	MISC		0.25	0.94	**0.27**	0.7		0.75	0.82	0.44	0.83
	SK		**0.26**	0.88	**0.15**	0.52		0.16	0.95	0.15	0.77
	AVG		**0.342**	0.842	**0.316**	**0.658**		0.448	0.878	0.408	0.756
EXP		CImg_MT7pts					DImg_MT7pts				
3	BCC		0.13	**0.96**	0.12	0.64		0.19	**0.98**	0.22	0.74
	NEV		0.46	0.77	0.56	0.69		0.71	0.7	0.73	0.79
	MEL	0.45	**0.65**	0.60	**0.46**	0.68	0.6	**0.42**	**0.93**	**0.51**	0.76
	MISC		0.23	0.94	0.26	0.7		0.8	0.83	0.48	0.87
	SK		0.11	**0.95**	0.1	0.56		**0.26**	0.95	**0.24**	0.82
	AVG		0.316	**0.844**	0.3	0.654		**0.476**	0.878	**0.436**	**0.796**

Figure 5.19 shows the multilabel confusion matrix for the single image combination of the 2ImgMd_CombFF_MT7pts. Both matrices look similar with the matrices of the third experiment 5.11. In both the clinical and dermoscopic matrices, the total number of predictions for the BCC and MISC increased and the total number of predictions for the NEV and MEL decreased. SK shows an increase in predictions in the clinical matrix, some of which were correctly classified samples, while the dermoscopic matrix shows the opposite. NEV is the class with the smallest changes in both matrices, while MEL shows the largest change in the clinical matrix, with a lower number of predictions, 10 of which were correctly classified samples.

The more focused models from the third experiment obtained higher global accuracy by focusing on the larger classes. This model did not perform as good as those, but the undersampled classes did benefit from the indirect influence from the other portions of the model. It is worth mentioning that the models performed similarly on the NEV class, it being the largest class.

5.12.2 Single Image and Metadata

The image and metadata combinations from the 2ImgMd_CombFF_MT7pts, obtains different results depending on the image type, as can be seen on Table 5.12.

The clinical image and metadata combination from the 2ImgMd_CombFF_MT7pts performs worse than its equivalent in most metric scores, obtaining lower global accuracy and lower average metric scores. The dermoscopic image and metadata combination from the 2ImgMd_CombFF_MT7pts performs better than its equivalent. Of the average metric scores,

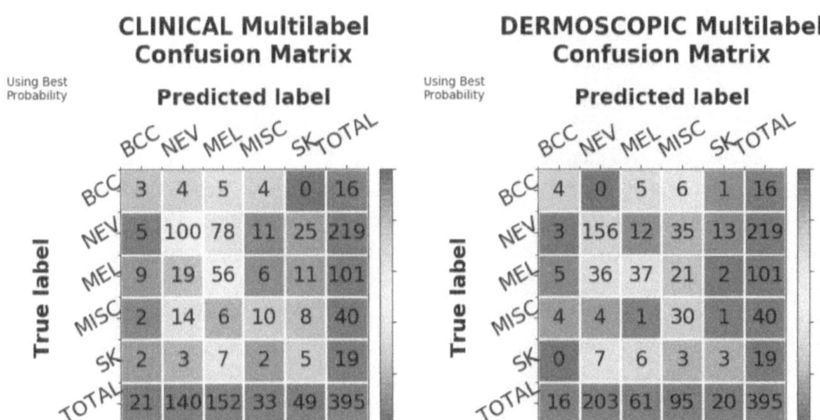

(a) Multilabel confusion matrix for the combination of the model trained on clinical images.

(b) Multilabel confusion matrix for the combination of the model trained on dermoscopic images.

Figure 5.19: Multilabel confusion matrices for the single image combination of the model of the eleventh experiment.

SEN obtains the largest increase, this is due to the higher SEN for the BCC, MEL and MISC classes. The performance of the NEV and SK classes improves slightly, with NEV obtaining a slightly higher AUROC score, while the SK class obtains slightly higher F1 and AUROC scores.

Table 5.12: Test metric scores for the 2ImgMd_CombFF_MT7pts (Single image and Metadata) (exp11) experiment and its equivalent, ImgMd_FF_MT7pts (exp8).

EXP		2ImgMd_CombFF_MT7pts (CImgMd)					2ImgMd_CombFF_MT7pts (DImgMd)				
		ACC	SEN	SPC	F1	AUROC	ACC	SEN	SPC	F1	AUROC
11	BCC	0.52	0.25	0.96	0.24	0.82	0.62	**0.44**	0.97	**0.42**	0.82
	NEV		0.57	0.8	0.65	0.75		0.71	**0.78**	0.75	0.83
	MEL		0.55	**0.71**	0.46	0.67		0.41	0.9	**0.48**	0.7
	MISC		0.35	0.92	0.34	0.73		**0.85**	0.82	**0.5**	0.89
	SK		0.32	0.93	0.23	0.69		0.26	0.97	**0.29**	0.78
	AVG		0.408	0.864	0.384	0.732		**0.534**	**0.888**	**0.488**	**0.804**
EXP		CImgMd_FF_MT7pts					DImgMd_FF_MT7pts				
8	BCC	0.56	**0.31**	**0.97**	**0.31**	0.86	0.61	0.38	**0.98**	0.39	0.81
	NEV		**0.61**	0.8	**0.69**	0.77		**0.76**	0.68	0.75	0.8
	MEL		**0.61**	0.7	**0.49**	0.68		0.35	**0.93**	0.45	0.75
	MISC		**0.4**	**0.95**	**0.44**	0.79		0.75	**0.85**	0.48	0.86
	SK		0.32	**0.94**	**0.26**	0.71		0.26	0.97	0.28	0.73
	AVG		**0.45**	**0.872**	**0.438**	**0.762**		0.5	0.882	0.47	0.79

Figure 5.20 shows the multilabel confusion matrix for the image and metadata combinations

from the 2ImgMd_CombFF_MT7pts. Like the Single image combination (res11i), the differences between these matrices and those of the eight experiment (Figure 5.16) are small. The clinical matrix (Figure 5.20a) shows a decrease in the true positives of most classes, with only the SK class reaching the same number of correctly classified samples. This occurs despite the increase in the number of predictions for the BCC, MISC and SK classes. The model decreased the umber of predictions for the NEV and MEL classes, but most of these were correctly classified samples. The dermoscopic matrix (Figure 5.20b) shows an increase in the number of predictions for the BCC, MEL and MISC classes, some of which are correctly classified samples, resolving in an increase in accuracy for the classes. The model lowers the number of predictions in the NEV class, some of which were correctly classified samples, but it does not change much the accuracy of the class. The model manages to have the same number of correctly classified samples in the SK class with one less prediction.

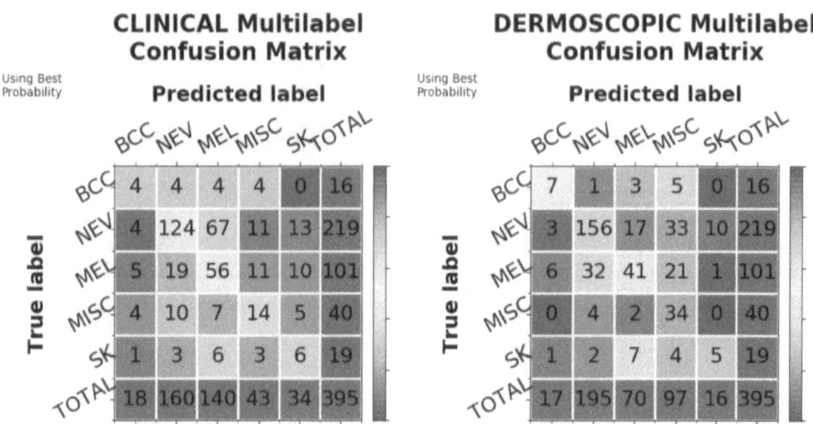

(a) Multilabel confusion matrix for the combination of the model trained on clinical images. (b) Multilabel confusion matrix for the combination of the model trained on dermoscopic images.

Figure 5.20: Multilabel confusion matrices for the single image and metadata combination of the model of the eleventh experiment.

The clinical image and metadata combination from the 2ImgMd_CombFF_MT7pts performed worse than its counterpart, with most of the metric scores being lower, while the dermoscopic image and metadata combination performed in the opposite direction, obtaining an overall better performance than the DImgMd_FF_MT7pts. Considering the conclusions from the tenth (concluded in res10) and eleventh (Single image) (concluded in res11i) experiments, it seems that this combination manage to benefit from indirect exposure to the clinical images through the other combinations. It seems that the model extracts better information from dermoscopic images, serving as a good foundation from which the other modalities can build upon. This theory is supported by the fact that every model trained on dermoscopic images from every experiment produced better results than the clinical counterpart.

5.12.3 Clinical Image, Dermoscopic image and Metadata

The all modalities combination from the 2ImgMd_CombFF_MT7pts produced a close result to that of the tenth experiment, 2ImgMd_FF_MT7pts (exp10). However, the tenth experiment obtained a better score for most of the average metric scores, despite obtaining the same global accuracy, with the all modalities combination acquiring better average SPC. Despite the average metric scores, there are some classes that do perform slightly better than the tenth experiment. NEV and MEL do obtain a higher F1-score but slightly worse AUROC. MISC obtained better AUROC and worse F1-score. The biggest difference occurs in the BCC and SK classes, where the eleventh experiment had a lower performance.

Table 5.13: Test metric scores for the 2ImgMd_CombFF_MT7pts (All Modalities) (exp11) experiment and its equivalent, 2ImgMd_FF_MT7pts (exp10).

EXP		2ImgMd_CombFF_MT7pts (2ImgMd)				
		ACC	SEN	SPC	F1	AUROC
11	BCC	0.65	0.31	0.97	0.29	0.7
	NEV		0.79	**0.72**	**0.79**	0.83
	MEL		**0.52**	0.86	**0.54**	0.74
	MISC		0.55	0.92	0.49	**0.85**
	SK		0.11	**0.98**	0.14	0.67
	AVG		0.456	**0.89**	0.45	0.758
EXP		2ImgMd_FF_MT7pts				
10	BCC	0.65	**0.44**	0.97	**0.41**	**0.73**
	NEV		**0.81**	0.68	0.78	**0.84**
	MEL		0.45	**0.89**	0.51	**0.75**
	MISC		**0.58**	0.92	**0.51**	0.84
	SK		**0.32**	0.97	**0.33**	**0.7**
	AVG		**0.52**	0.886	**0.508**	**0.772**

Figure 5.21 shows the multilabel confusion matrix and the ROC curves of the all modalities combination of the 2ImgMd_CombFF_MT7pts. The matrix, seen in Figure 5.21a, shows the BCC class with a lower number of correctly classified samples, but maintaining the same number of predictions. MISC has a decrease in predictions and correctly classified samples of one, while SK lowers both considerably. NEV also has a lower number of predictions, some of which were correctly classified samples. The MEL class has an increase in the number of predictions, most of which are correctly classified samples, increasing the accuracy of the class.

The ROC curves shown in Figure 5.21b indicate a similar performance for the MISC and NEV classes, with MEL and SK obtaining lower AUROC and the performance on the BCC class starting to lower sooner.

Performing several combinations of modalities in the same model allows for each of the various

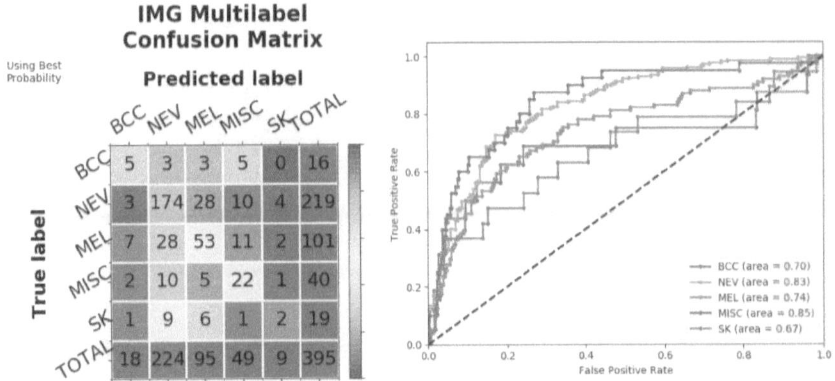

(a) Multilabel confusion matrix for the combin-(b) ROC curves for the model trained on all modalities.
ation of the model trained on clinical images.

Figure 5.21: Multilabel confusion matrices for the clinical image, dermoscopic image and metadata combination of the model of the eleventh experiment.

combinations to be exposed indirectly to the modalities that they do not include. This makes it so that each combination does not fit to its best, but it does allow a small influence from the missing modalities. This is reflected in the single image combinations and the dermoscopic and metadata combination were there was a better performance in the BCC class, typically seen when the model is allowed to use the excluded modalities. Cases such as the dermoscopic image and metadata combination that were able to reach better results in this kind of model are possible, but do not seem to be the norm, as all the other combinations did not improve, while the all modalities combination only achieved similar global accuracy, obtaining lower scores in most of the average metric scores. As such it seems that performing these combinations in a single model does not necessarily improve the result, only occasionally having the better performing combination.

5.13 Summary

5.13.1 Baseline

Throughout this chapter, several results were presented. The first experiment (res1) provided a baseline for the next experiments to compare to.

5.13.2   Class-fusion and feature-fusion.

The second experiment (res2) introduces metadata through class-fusion, improving the performance of the models on the BCC class, but with a considerable negative effect on the performance
of the larger classes of NEV and MEL. The seventh experiment (res7) fused images with
metadata through feature-fusion, not increasing as much the performance over the BCC class as
the class-fusion, but substantially reducing the negative impact on the larger classes, and as such
obtaining higher global accuracy and higher average metric scores.

5.13.3   Multitasking

The third experiment (res3) introduced multitasking of the categories of the 7-point checklist,
this produced a slight increase in the performance of the larger classes, i.e. the NEV and MEL
classes. The fourth experiment (res4), introduced transfer learning to the fusion with metadata,
this reduced the negative effect that metadata brought on the larger classes, while still improving
the performance of the BCC class. The fifth experiment (res5) attempted to multitask with
metadata, a categorical modality that can be fused with the images, and, much like when it is
fused with images, a reduced improvement to the performance in the BCC class is present, as
well as the clinical model generally improving its performance in the larger classes, while the
dermoscopic model worsened the performance in the larger classes. Lastly the sixth experiment
(res6) applied transfer learning with this knowledge, where it did provide a general improvement
on the performance of both models, but it did not obtain results as good as the transfer learning
from the multitask of the 7-points.

5.13.4   Multitasking and multimodality

The eight experiment (res8) applied multitasking to the feature-fusion, producing better results
than either class-fusion or feature-fusion.

The ninth experiment (res9) fused both image types, seeing an increase in the performance
on BCC over the image-only models of the third experiment, improving the performance of the
MISC to the same level as the dermoscopic models and generally improving the performance
over both the NEV and MEL classes.

5.13.5   Multitasking and all modalities

The tenth experiment (res10) sees the fusion of all of the available modalities, producing the
best results in from these experiments.

Lastly, the eleventh experiment (res11) joins the third, eight and tenth models in a single
model. This model with various combinations of modalities only produce better results in one of

its combinations, the dermoscopic image and metadata, while the other combinations performing worse than the isolated models. It took a longer time to train this larger model than any of the individual models. However, if it is compared with the added times of each of the individual models it would finish training considerably faster. Considering that the results obtained from the combination model are similar, if slightly lower, than the focused model, this combination model might be a good way to investigate various possibilities at the same time.

Chapter 6

Conclusion

In this chapter the conclusions are presented, along with the main contributions as well as some research directions to extend the work. The conclusions are presented in Section 6.1, with the main contributions following in Section 6.2, while the encountered limitations and future work are presented in Section 6.3.

6.1   Conclusions

The field of dermoscopy raised significant interest, and there are datasets with various modalities, each containing valuable information to aid in the correct classification of cancerous skin lesions. This work investigates the efficacy of each modality used for training a CNN. Other works conducted in this thesis investigate the application of various techniques to improve the classification, as well as the viability of a simple network for feature extraction from images, fusion of features and classification. As such, several experiments were carried out to compare the modalities available and observe if the application of the techniques improves the classification process. These experiments are performed by a simple network, each model obtaining small improvements in the results over the previous experiment. The results obtained were lower than those reported in the literature [44, 46, 75], this is expected as a simpler network, without extensive pre-training, was utilized. The aim of this thesis is to investigate the impact of using various modalities rather than achieving a high performance classification model. Several conclusions are extracted from these experiments.

The baseline created in the first (exp1) experiment shows that the results obtained by the model trained on dermoscopic images were considerably higher than those obtained by the model trained on clinical images, as is seen on Table 5.1. This leads to the conclusion that the dermoscopic images contain more useful information than the clinical images.

The results of the second (exp2) and seventh (exp7) experiments point to the feature fusion is mitigating the negative effect of an un-ballanced dataset, while the class-fusion produced a heavy bias for the Basal Cell Carcinoma (BCC), which decreased the performance of the other classes with more samples. As such the feature-fusion seems to be a better approach to fusing data.

The third (exp3) and fifth (exp5) experiments indicate that multitasking introduces an indirect influence the model from the other modalities, resulting in smaller impacts from the exposure (compared to fusing the modalities). The multitasking of the categories of the 7-points lead to a small increase in the performance of the models in the Nevus (NEV) and Seborrheic Keratosis (SK) classes, while multitasking the metadata increased slightly the performance of the models over the BCC class. The increases in performance were obtained with reduced results from other classes, although these varied depending on the model and multitasking. Despite the multitasking of the categories of the 7-points increased the performance of the models for the classes with more samples, only the model trained on dermoscopic images has scored a higher accuracy, average Sensitivity (SEN) and average F1-score. The model trained on clinical images obtained higher global accuracy and average Specificity (SPC) and average F1-score by multitasking the metadata. This indicates that the model trained on clinical images benefits more from exposure to categorical metadata such as location, elevation and sex. As metadata can be used as input data, with a stronger impact over the final output, it is preferable to multitask the categories of the 7-points over the multitasking of metadata.

The fourth (exp4) and sixth (exp6) experiments show the results of pre-training the model on some modalities first. Transfer learning is used to preserve the knowledge obtained, while other modalities are multitasked. This enables the use of modalities both as output and later as input. Thanks to the way the models were trained, the fusions produced considerably better results than just class-fusion. The model trained on dermoscopic images did not obtain lower global accuracy and average metric scores than the baseline, when compared with the class-fusion model. In fact, the transfer learning using the multitasking of the categories of the 7-points produced higher global accuracy and average metric scores than either the other transfer learning models or the baseline. This result, in addition to dermoscopic images containing more information, as well as the results from fusing with metadata being generally lower, indicates that the available metadata is not easily fused with dermoscopic images. This shows that there can be modalities that do not fuse easily with others, causing a reduction in the performance of the a model, which leads to lower results. For these cases, sequentially training the model on the modalities, as opposed to training the model using various modalities at the same time, can be a good alternative.

The third (exp3) and eighth (exp8) experiments demonstrate that multitasking provides a general increase of the results, while the fifth (exp5) experiment shows that the increase from the technique is due to multitasking the categories of the 7-points specifically. In addition, the eighth (exp8) experiment also shows that the effects from multitasking the categories of the 7-points can balance the effects of fusing with the metadata, obtaining higher performance in all of NEV, Melanoma (MEL) and BCC classes from the models. As such the usage of multitasking is encouraged.

The ninth (exp9) and tenth (exp10) experiments show that the usage of multiple modalities produce higher results than relying solely on each modality. This is despite the considerably lower results from the models trained on clinical images and the usage of a simple architecture.

As such using multiple modalities is advised, especially since lower results can be due to an improper fusion method, as is observed in the models trained on dermoscopic images of the second (exp2) and fourth (exp4) experiments.

Lastly, the eleventh (exp11) experiment, comparing with the eighth (exp8), ninth (exp9) and tenth (exp10) experiments, shows that multitasking a large number of learning tasks reduces the performances for each of the learning tasks. This results in generally lower results, when compared with the more focused models. There are occurrences, such as the combination of dermoscopic image and metadata from the eleventh experiment, that obtained higher results than its equivalent, as is seen in Table 5.12. However, the remaining combinations obtained lower results than their equivalents, including the best performing combination of all modalities. As such, it is more reliable to utilize a focused model to obtain the best results.

Few other papers utilized the same dataset, and those that did, also added data from other sources. Regardless, our best results, obtained in the tenth experiment (exp10), are not the best in the literature, as can be seen in Table 6.1. With the average AUROC having 0.092 score difference from the closest in [75], SEN having 0.084 score difference from the closest in [44] and SPC having 0.024 score difference from the closest in [44]. This is due to the usage of a simpler network. In [75] a classical approach is utilized. With considerable effort put to identify several areas of the lesion and extracting a variety of features from each of the areas. It has the lowest Area under the receiver operating characteristic (AUROC) among the papers in Table 6.1. The other two papers utilize some form of Deep Neural Network (DNN) to extract features. The networks utilized are larger and pre-trained utilizing transfer learning, therefore obtaining higher results. The results obtained in [44] are the most relevant, as their methodology was adapted in this work. All of our results are lower, with the AUROC and SEN being $\approx 13.8\%$ lower and SPC being $\approx 2.6\%$ lower.

Table 6.1: Results of other papers and our best result
(2ImgMd_FF_MT7pts exp10).

Paper	Dataset	AUROC	SEN	SPC
[75]	EDRA + other	0.864		
[46]	EDRA + other	0.911	0.853	0.940
[44]	EDRA	0.896	0.604	0.910
ours (2ImgMd_FF_MT7pts exp10)	EDRA	0.772	0.520	0.886

This result, however, does not show that a simpler network is not viable. The simplicity enables for quicker testing, allowing for experimenting of other ideas and provides a proof of concept. These ideas can then be integrated in a larger network, where its capacity to both train to a higher degree and extract better features would lead to acquiring better results.